Textbook of Developmental Paediatrics

Dedicated
Op. cit. to B.P. and W.A.M.
and
to Dr Richard Sutton and Mrs Ann Ingram, who have kept me
well enough to write this book.

Original line drawings
by Jane Upton

For Churchill Livingstone

Publisher: Georgina Bentliff
Project Editor: Lucy Gardner
Copy Editors: Neil Pakenham-Walsh and Isabel Kirkwood
Indexer: Brian Armitage
Production Controller: Mark Sanderson
Sales Promotion Executive: Kathy Crawford

Textbook of
Developmental Paediatrics

Margaret Pollak MD MB BS FRCGP DObst RCOG

Reader Emeritus in Developmental and Educational Paediatrics, University of London; Honorary Research Fellow, King's College Hospital Medical School, London; Formerly Medical Director, Sir Wilfrid Sheldon Children's Centre and Honorary Consultant Paediatrician, Department of Child Health, King's College Hospital, London

CHURCHILL LIVINGSTONE
EDINBURGH LONDON MADRID MELBOURNE NEW YORK AND TOKYO 1993

CHURCHILL LIVINGSTONE
Medical Division of Longman Group UK Limited

Distributed in the United States of America by Churchill
Livingstone Inc., 650 Avenue of the Americas, New York,
N.Y. 10011, and by associated companies, branches and
representatives throughout the world.

First published 1993

ISBN 0-443-04169-5

British Library Cataloguing in Publication Data
A catalogue record for this book is available from the British
Library.

Library of Congress Cataloging in Publication Data
Pollak, Margaret.
    Textbook of developmental paediatrics / Margaret Pollak.
        p.   cm.
    Includes index.
    ISBN 0-443-04169-5
    1. Child development.   2. Child psychology.   3. Child
development deviations.   I. Title.
    (DNLM: 1. Child Development. WS 105 P769t)
RJ47.5.P65 1993
618.92--dc20
DNLM/DLC
for Library of Congress   92–22842
                                                CIP

Produced by Longman Singapore Publishers (Pte) Ltd
Printed in Singapore

Preface

Any medical textbook will blend published scientific findings with clinical experience. When I first began to learn my craft, information in books was hard to come by. It was – and largely still is – a case of reading journals, assimilating patients' records and extrapolating from allied books. This book is a first attempt to bring knowledge, currently diverse, together in one book. There will be sins and omissions, but perhaps it will provide the foundation upon which others can build.

I am neither feminist nor male chauvinist. The English language, having no neuter, does not allow pronouns to apply to both genders. I will not consider the impersonal 'it'. After long thought, I have succumbed to the grammatical 'he'. I hope my fellow females will forgive me.

London, 1993   M.P.

Acknowledgements

I have pleasure in acknowledging the debt owed to:
    Arnold Gesell, whose books were an inspiration and whose writings
    kindled an interest in the subject,
    Mary Sheridan, whose pupil I was fortunate to be,
    to all the children and parents whom I have had the privilege of
    knowing.

M.P.

Contents

1. Developmental paediatrics   1

2. Development   19

3. Factors which affect development   47

4. History-taking and medical examination   81

5. Developmental examination   115

6. Motor development   145

7. Personalsocial development   195

8. Adaptive development   241

9. Language development   275

10. Play and learning   323

11. Hearing   371

12. Vision   413

13. Handicapped children   459

14. Diagnosis, treatment and care   505

15. The practice of developmental paediatrics   549

Index   567

main priority is to deal with the everyday, individual presentation of development. Paediatrics is concerned with the whole child. Since every child is growing and developing, paediatricians need to know whether the current developmental state is normal, average or abnormal; whether retarded or advanced, i.e. make a developmental diagnosis. In addition, there is the need to know what are the factors which can operate to affect development — for better or worse — and whether clinicians are in a position to manipulate any of these factors to the child's benefit. Paediatricians, being doctors, also need to know abnormal as well as delayed development and how disease and medical conditions may mar development. Thus for the paediatrician child development is the norm against which any particular child can be matched and abnormal development is of as much concern as normal.

REFERENCES

Ames L B 1989 Arnold Gesell: themes of his work. Human Sciences Press, New York
Apley J 1978 Ronald Charles MacKeith. In : Apley J (ed) Care of handicapped child. A Festschrift for Ronald MacKeith. Clinics in Developmental Medicine 67. Spastics International Medical Publications/ Heinemann Medical Books, London, pp 1–9
Aries P 1962 Centuries of childhood: a social history of family life. Vintage Books, New York
Bandura A, Walters R H 1963 Social learning and personality development. Holt, New York
Bandura A 1977 Social learning theory. Prentice–Hall, Englewood Cliffs, New Jersey
Bax M C O, Whitmore K 1990 Controversy: reviews of a book, Health for all children. Archives of Disease in Childhood 65: 141–142
Bayley N 1933 Mental growth during the first three years. Genetic Psychology Monograph 14: 1
Binet A, Simon T 1916 The development of intelligence in children. Williams & Wilkins, Baltimore
Bowlby J 1969 Attachment and loss, vol 1. Basic Books, New York
Central Health Services Council 1967 Child welfare centres: Report of sub-committee of standing medical advisory committee of Council (Sheldon Report)
Cohen S 1966 The problem of Piaget's child. Teachers College Record 68: 211–218
Darwin C 1859 The origin of species, 1st edn.
Darwin C 1872 The expression of the emotions in man and animals. Murray, London, 1965 edn. University of Chicago Press, Chicago
Darwin C 1877 A biographical sketch of an infant. Mind 285–294
De Mause L 1974 The history of childhood. Souvenir Press
Egan D 1989 Personal communication
Erikson E H 1964 Insight and responsibility. Norton, New York
Erikson E H 1967 Childhood and society. Penguin, Harmondsworth
Estes B W 1972 Some mathematical and logical concepts in children. In: Behrens H, Maynard G (eds) The changing child. Scott and Foresman, Glenview, Illinois
Frankenburg W K, Dodds J B 1967 The Denver developmental screening test. Journal of Pediatrics 71: 181
Gesell A 1922 Mental and physical correspondence in twins. Scientific Monthly 14: 305–344
Gesell A 1925 Developmental diagnosis in infancy. Boston Medical and Surgical Journal 192: 1058–1064
Gesell A, Amatruda C S 1941 Developmental diagnosis: normal and abnormal child development. Harper & Row, New York
Gesell A 1941 Developmental diagnosis. Hoeber Medical Division

Gesell A, Amatruda C S 1947 Developmental diagnosis: normal and abnormal child development. Harper & Row, New York

Gesell A 1948 The mental growth of the preschool child. Harper & Row, New York

Gesell A 1949 The first five years of life. Methuen, London

Gesell A, Amatruda C S 1965 Developmental diagnosis: normal and abnormal child development, 2nd edn. Hoeber/Harper & Row, New York

Goldberg S 1966 Probability judgements by preschool children: task conditions and performance. Child Development 37: 157–167

Griffiths R 1954 The abilities of babies. University of London Press, London

Hall D M B, Baird G 1986 Developmental tests and scales. Archives of Disease in Childhood 61: 213–215

Illingworth R S 1960 The development of the infant and young child: normal and abnormal, 1st edn. Churchill Livingstone, Edinburgh

Illingworth R S 1981 Your child's development in the first five years. (Patient's handbook.) Churchill Livingstone, Edinburgh

Illingworth R S 1982 Basic developmental screening: 0–2 years, 3rd edn. Blackwell Scientific Publications, Oxford

Illingworth R S 1987 The development of the infant and young child: normal and abnormal, 9th edn. Churchill Livingstone, Edinburgh

Inhelder B 1944 Le diagnostique du raisinnement chez les debiles mentaux. Delachaux et Niestle, Neuchatel

Isaacs S 1933a Intellectual growth in children. Routledge and Kegan Paul, London

Isaacs S 1933b Social development of children. Routledge and Kegan Paul, London

Joint Working Party on Child Health Surveillance 1989 In: Hall D M B (ed) Health for all children. Oxford University Press, Oxford

Keating D P, Clark L V 1980 Development of physical and social reasoning in adolescence. Developmental Psychology 11: 531–532

Kennell J H, Jerauld R, Wolfe H et al 1974 Maternal behaviour one year after early and extended post-partum contact. Developmental Medicine and Child Neurology 16: 172–179

Knobloch H, Pasamanick B 1974 Developmental diagnosis. Harper & Row, New York

Lansdown R 1984 Child development. Heinemann, London

Pollock L A 1983 Forgotten Children: parent–child relations from 1500–1900. Cambridge University Press, Cambridge

Polnay L 1989 Child health surveillance. New report highlights value of parental observations. British Medical Journal 299: 1351–1352

Preyer W 1881 The mind of the child.

Rutter M 1980 Scientific foundations of developmental psychiatry. Heinemann, London

Serebriakoff V 1990 Educating the intelligent child. Mensa Publications

Sheridan M D 1978 The fashioning of a human life-style. Child: Care, Health and Development 4: 425–429

Skinner B F 1957 Verbal behaviour. Appleton–Century–Crofts, New York

Touwen B C L, Prechtl H F R 1970 The neurological examination of the child with minor nervous dysfunction. Clinics in Developmental Medicine 38. Spastics International Medical Publications/Heinemann Medical Books, London

Weikart D P 1972 Relationship of curriculum, teaching and learning in preschool education. In: Stanley J C (ed) Preschool programs for the disadvantaged. Johns Hopkins University Press, Baltimore

Winnicott D W 1957 The child and the outside world. Basic Books, New York

2. Development

The child is father of the Man

William Wordsworth

What is development? Whilst the purist may say human beings continue to develop all their lives, generally development is the characteristic which distinguishes children from adults. Normal children do not remain static in physical and mental growth or development, whilst these changes are minimal in the adult. Development is divided into the physiological, anatomical and behavioural and each subdivision depends to a varying degree upon the other. Thus factors affecting the development of one are likely to impinge upon the development of another.

Many branches of medicine are concerned with one system or even one organ of the human body. Paediatrics is concerned with a whole being, namely, a child. Development characterizes this child. Thus paediatrics is concerned with development in *all* subdivisions, piecing them together to study the whole. Furthermore, a study of development involves the subnormal, the normal and the superior but no diagnosis of an abnormal state can be made without a wide knowledge of what is normal in the same way that clinical medicine requires a knowledge of the range of normality. Therefore the making of any developmental diagnosis, and especially a differential diagnosis, lies within the realms of clinical paediatrics.

An important question is how development occurs. A plethora of theories of development was noted in Chapter 1. The fact that so many theories abound suggests that no single one is entirely satisfactory and, in clinical practice, this is true. The most common reason is that the majority of theories are concerned with only one, or possibly two, parameters of development. No single theory concerns itself with enmeshing of each and every parameter into a whole. Yet, to make a comprehensive developmental diagnosis this is necessary. It might be argued that this is one of the primary tasks of developmental paediatrics.

PARAMETERS OF DEVELOPMENT

Just as no single theory adequately answers the whole of development so no single system of developmental assessment is complete.

19

The most comprehensive system is that of Gesell whose subdivisions of development are: Motor; Personalsocial; Language; Adaptive.

One of the advantages of these subdivisions is that the parameter 'personalsocial development' encompasses both the individual's development of himself, his personality and attitudes *together with* his social development in relation to others. A second advantage is the separation of nonverbal skills (adaptive development) from motor development (sic). A third advantage is the measuring from the very earliest years of language and nonverbal skills so when the child is older these can be merged to accord with IQ tests, the best of which always have a verbal and nonverbal (or performance) component.

An estimate of verbal and nonverbal skills is invaluable when making a differential diagnosis of development. One example is a deaf child who may have poor language development but, if of normal intelligence, will have average nonverbal skills. If nonverbal skills are not assessed in addition to language, it is impossible to differentiate between language delay and mental retardation. A second example is a mentally retarded child whose language and nonverbal skills are low but whose language is comparatively higher than nonverbal skills if he lives in a very stimulating environment, language being more susceptible to the environment than are nonverbal skills. (A further refinement is that expressive language may be superior to comprehension — see Ch. 10). In this case, the differential diagnosis between delayed language and global retardation is impossible unless both verbal and nonverbal skills are assessed.

Several schemes of developmental assessment, particularly the Denver (Frankenburg et al 1967), the Bayley Scales (Bayley 1969) and the Griffiths Mental Development Scales (Griffiths 1970) are based on Gesell's schemata. They are described in Chapter 5.

These are some of the advantages of using Gesell scales. A disadvantage is that sensory development is not included. It is essential to examine hearing and vision, not only for normality or pathology but also for developmental levels. For example, socially disadvantaged children, thought to be deaf, responded accurately to hearing tests when those suitable for a younger age group were used (Pollak 1972). They were not socially experienced or mature enough to undertake hearing tests suitable for their own age group. This is a good example of the need to know the meaning of developmental status as well as normal acuity.

In the UK, developmental assessments have been much influenced by the work of Mary Sheridan who subdivided development into the following parameters: Posture and Large Movements; Vision and Fine Movements; Hearing and Speech; Social Behaviour and Play.

As a result of Mary Sheridan's influence many developmental surveillance and assessment programmes are based on these parameters. Unfortunately, however, there are problems in using these subdivisions.

Although eye-motor coordination is particularly important during the first year of life and this could justify assessment of fine manipulation and vision together during the first year, in reality, the development of fine manipulation and vision each warrant separate study. Hearing certainly affects the development of language but the development of language is an extremely important and complicated parameter of development which requires independent assessment and it is important to know and understand the development of hearing separately from linguistic skills.

Social development as a developmental parameter implies interaction with other humans and does not take into account the development of a child's individual personality and emotional growth which is implicit in Gesell's personalsocial development parameter.

Nonverbal skills are not studied as a separate parameter although some are included in the assessment of fine motor and vision skills. However, whilst the ability to place one brick upon another and release is a skill of fine manipulation and eye-motor coordination, the ability to copy a 'house' is a skill of a higher order (Fig. 2.1). It is exactly at this stage of brick play that mentally retarded children become delayed and adaptive development needs assessing separately from fine motor and vision skills to demonstrate this. Performance with a formboard demonstrates the same point. The putting of a round shape into a round hole is a motor skill. But watch a child faced with a three-shape formboard. Some children pick up a shape and haplessly try to force it into any hole (motor skill). Some pick it up and immediately place it in the correct hole (good eye-motor coordination). Yet others will pick up the shape, examine it visually, scan the shapes of all the holes and place it in the correct hole. What might have been thought an instinctive motor skill has, by the third method, been transformed into an intellectual exercise.

A comprehensive developmental assessment will include a study of the following developmental parameters:

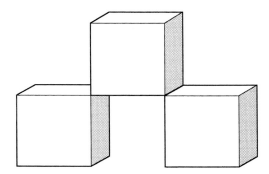

Fig. 2.1   A 'house' of three 1-inch bricks.

- Physical growth.
- Motor development — gross and fine manipulation, balance and movement.
- Personalsocial development.
- Adaptive (or nonverbal) development.
- Communication and language development.
- Learning.
- Hearing.
- Vision.

In school-age children language and adaptive development can be combined to give a score of IQ. However, if language and adaptive development are retained separately they provide information about each parameter not conveyed by the IQ. This may be important in children with learning difficulties.

PHYSICAL GROWTH

Growth infers increase in size but in some organs also involves development of function, including multiplication and differentiation of cells, pattern formation and change in form. It is common practice to measure the height, weight and head circumferences as measures of growth and record these on centile charts (see Ch. 4). After the first year of life, growth in length during the next 10 years occurs in an orderly fashion although different organs grow at different rates. 'The whole affair is quite extraordinarily regular' (Tanner 1956). This regularity allows prediction of adult height from the current height and this estimate is likely to be correct to within 5 cm (Tanner 1975). Because of the regularity of the growing process, if a child is falling below his previous percentile there is likely to be a reason for it which should be sought. This prediction does *not* apply during adolescence because of the growth spurt. The final height is unrelated to whether the spurt comes early or late (Tanner 1970). Prediction also does not apply during the first months of life because babies, especially those born small, are likely to catch up and cross onto higher percentiles.

A rule of thumb for *weight* is that it is likely to be doubled by 5 months and tripled by the first birthday whilst *height* is likely to increase by about 25 cm in the first year and be almost half full adult height by 2 years (Bee 1981).

Head circumference cannot be equated with brain growth. The increase in head circumference takes an upward spurt in the 2–6 months following birth and there is another spurt from age 2–4 years. In between these times the curve is more linear. Brain growth, unlike circumference, continues in a more orderly fashion. During the antenatal period the brain grows in an extremely rapid manner so that at birth it is already 25% of its adult weight (Dobbing et al 1978). The head of a newborn is much larger in proportion to the body than in adulthood (Fig. 2.2). At birth the midbrain is the most developed part of the brain. The cortex increases in cell number and connections and is approximately half completed by 6 months of age and three-quarters by 2 years. By 6 months of age, therefore, the cortex begins its domination. This can explain the disappearance of some of the reflexes seen in the newborn. The growth of the cortex is by no means even. For example, areas dealing with hearing and vision are well developed at birth; motor development takes place soon afterwards whilst higher cognitive functions come later and explain what a baby can achieve at any particular age. Myelinization, even of the spinal cord, is not complete at birth but, during the ensuing months, the sheathing of the spinal cord and other nerves proceeds rapidly and is almost complete by 2 years of age whilst myelinization and growth of connective tissue of the brain continues for longer, sometimes into adolescence. Concurrently with the closure of the neural tube, some neurons of the motor horn cells of the spinal cord and motor nuclei of the brain stem are formed whilst others (especially in the cerebellum, olfactory bulb and hippocampus) are produced after birth. A knowledge of neurogenesis is helpful in the understanding of early developmental processes and possible symptoms in some congenital malformations (Rodier 1980).

Bones grow by hardening and increasing in size. The skull bones develop from several into one and grow over the soft fontanelles but some bones increase in number, e.g. hands, wrists, feet and ankles. At birth cardiac output (per kg body weight) is about three times that of an adult due to a considerably higher oxygen consumption. It decreases soon afterwards. Respiratory rate decreases with age: peak flow increases but does not reach adult flow rate until the teens.

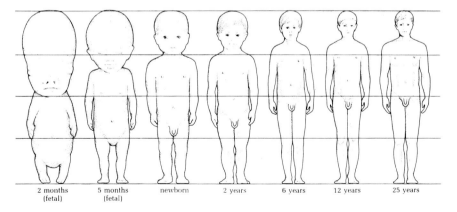

| 2 months (fetal) | 5 months (fetal) | newborn | 2 years | 6 years | 12 years | 25 years |

Fig. 2.2 Changes in proportions of the human body. (From Schaffer D R 1985 Developmental psychology. Brooks/Cole, Monterey, California)

The development of the immunological system, which involves the production of antibodies, destruction of infections and resistance to disease, is very complicated and readers are referred to textbooks on the subject. The immediate neonatal period is low in immunoglobulins (except IgG) because they do not cross the placental barrier and the baby has not yet developed his own. The digestive system is also subject to development. In general, the important facts are that babies during the early months absorb proteins well but have difficulty with starch, fat and sometimes sugar digestion.

Hormone production changes during childhood. The thyroid growth hormones and testosterone are present in prenatal life. Growth postnatally is essentially governed by the thyroid and pituitary glands until adolescence when the adrenal and sex hormones will exert their effects on pubertal growth.

Disorders of growth vary according to the organ involved. For example, children with myelomeningocele have a growth defect which leads to short stature (Rosenblum et al 1983). *Failure to thrive* is a common presenting problem in early infancy accounting for 5% of hospital admissions to a paediatric ward during one year. When due to an organic abnormality, failure to thrive is likely to present early and be accompanied by breathlessness in cardiac abnormalities or vomiting and diarrhoea in gastrointestinal disorders. Most cases of failure to thrive are not due to organic abnormality. Deprivational dwarfism (Gardner 1972) has been described in children who are adequately fed but emotionally starved. Oral-motor abnormality or immaturity has been described in this type of failure (Mathisen et al 1989).

Children who are malnourished grow either slowly or not at all but when malnourishment is neither prolonged nor severe and diet improved, they grow more quickly than normal — 'catch up growth' (Tanner 1978). This phenomenon has been described after long-term fostercare which followed child abuse (King et al 1985).

Growth may be *abnormal*. For example, muscles and limbs may fail to grow in upper and lower motor neurone diseases although more likely in the latter. Both conditions are associated with a poor general physique. Although unusual, growth may be *enhanced* and is seen in some cases of cerebral tumours and hydrocephalus and has been reported, uncommonly, following tuberculous meningitis (Holt 1980). *Obesity*, defined as 20% over expected weight for sex and height, is commonly multifactorial. It occurs in certain medical conditions of which lesions of the hypothalamus and the Prader-Willi syndrome are the most common.

There is little agreement as to the time interval which should be allowed for low birthweight and small-for-dates babies to catch up, i.e. how long to make allowance. The American Academy of Pediatrics recommends that corrections should be made until 2 years of age. However, Nelson et al (1985) suggest that correction may be needed up to 3 years of age.

Illingworth (1987) declines to set guidelines. In practice, the time generally appears to be much less.

MOTOR DEVELOPMENT

Motor development is subdivided into gross motor development and fine manipulation.

Gross motor development

This is concerned with how children use their body, such as posture, prehension, balance and movement. A baby advances from a head that sags to one over which he has complete control. He develops sitting, rolling over, crawling, pulling to stand, standing and walking. Standing on one leg, running, jumping, skipping, going up stairs, riding a bicycle, etc. are all refinements of these basic skills and movements. Some skills are developed in parallel: he is learning to sit, to move in prone and pull to supine at more or less the same time. Babies also learn to change from one posture to another and to move. Some early movements and other motor functions are initially reflex but develop, through a series of phases of ever increasing efficiency, towards the skilful but eventually automatic selection of muscles and movements required to perform a task. This can only be achieved by coordination of the central nervous system, nerves and muscles. Gesell believed that motor development was almost entirely a matter of maturation and that of the central nervous system in particular. He placed reliance for his theory on a pair of twins. One was given practice in acquiring a motor skill whilst the other was not. The second twin quickly caught up after very little practice (Gesell & Thompson 1929). It is unlikely that maturation is the whole picture. When the ability to perform a task has been acquired, awareness, selection and the wish to perform the skill are still required in order to achieve it.

Development in the motor parameter involves speed. Older children are quicker than younger children at performing a task due to increased skill in performance. A so-called clumsy or overactive child may appear, at first sight, to be very quick but on closer observation is seen to be impulsive rather than efficiently fast.

Gross motor development is subject to most of the rules of development outlined in Chapter 1, i.e. goes through well defined *stages*. We cannot run before we can walk. Development is *cephalo-caudal and proximodistal*. A baby develops head control before he can sit and lifts his chest off a couch before he can use his arms. Development of hand and finger movements are refinements of proximodistal development.

Ball playing can be used as an example of *differentiation* — or going from the general to the specific. Gradually, learning and practice can improve performance to ever increasing definition and sophistication.

When catching a ball, the 2-year-old holds out both hands, the whole body is involved and he can only catch a big ball. He has not yet developed the eye-motor coordination of measuring the distance and speed of the ball and often closes his eyes to receive the ball. By 5 years he can catch a much smaller ball which is bounced to him with a two-hand catch free of his body and by 9 years he can catch a tennis ball in one outstretched hand (Stott et al 1972). To reach this stage has taken time, phases have been passed and finally maturity is reached.

Fine manipulation

The ability to use hands, fingers and thumbs with ever increasing agility and precision are skills acquired later than some gross motor skills, head control in particular, and has implications for pathological conditions in which adequate head control is never acquired. Development of fine manipulation is helped by the ability to sit up but hampered by the prone position and crawling. Sitting and rolling over to prone are movements which are acquired at the same time. Thus, in the sitting position hands are free and when free can reach out, grasp and release objects. The development of fine manipulation is an important skill which differentiates man from most animals. The baby begins to focus on arm's length distance just at the time he begins to grasp objects with outstretched hands, visual focal length coinciding with the stage of motor development. Motor development also relies upon good kinaesthetic sense and the development of perception. Motor development may be subnormal, normal, superior or abnormal. Changes from normal occur in gross and fine skills but fine manipulation being the more advanced skill is the more often affected.

Subnormal motor development implies that the stages are normal but delayed. For example, many mentally retarded children are delayed in sitting and walking but in the absence of a motor condition, motor development is often the least delayed parameter. The motor delay is often due to an associated hypotonia. Blind babies are usually late in passing their early motor milestones, reflecting the influence of kinaesthetic sense on motor development. There have been several reports of the superior or, more accurately, advanced early motor development of negro babies, an advance which later slows down, but the athletic prowess of the negro race is famed.

Abnormal motor development is seen in disorders of movement and posture of which cerebral palsy is the most common. Muscular dystrophy and spina bifida are other examples. Children with cerebral palsy show both abnormal and late motor development. Abnormality of motor development is seen when a baby is locked in one developmental stage and does not develop in another — he can sit, but cannot roll over and crawl. Another example is when arm and leg patterns do not match. The persistence of reflexes, e.g. the Moro, TNR and grasp, which usually disappear, are examples of abnormal motor development in cerebral palsy.

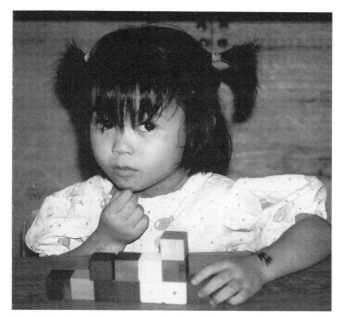

Fig. 2.8 A south Vietnamese girl in a refugee camp in Hong Kong.

child, whose language is poor, will undertake these tests at age-appropriate levels. A child with language delay will also perform at age level. Most children with severe language disorders have normal nonverbal skills until 4 – 5 years of age or, even if not age-appropriate, their achievement will exceed their linguistic skills. On the other hand, mentally retarded children, especially if living in a stimulating home, have higher levels in language development than nonverbal skills. Assessment of children's scores in nonverbal development thus makes a differential diagnosis possible.

DEVELOPMENT OF COMMUNICATION

Although no-one could deny that animals can communicate with each other and Washoe, the chimpanzee, is said to have invented three-word sentences (Gardner et al 1974), the development of language is considered to be man's highest function and distinguishes man from animals.

However, this parameter of development includes very much more than the acquisition of language. Communication includes nonverbal behaviour such as facial expression, gesture and postural movements as well as verbal skills. Hearing and communication are intertwined. A new baby is bombarded with sounds which he needs to hear and understand. Soon, he tries out sounds of his own which he understands and uses for self expression. A higher intellectual function is to analyse both comprehended and expressed language. Communication begins at birth, babies being extremely adroit at recognizing their mother's voice in distinction to other female voices (DeCasper et al 1980). Babbling occurs by 3–4 months of age and communication becomes a social exercise with the baby and mother taking turns to communicate. Imitation follows and is succeeded by words which are increasingly used with meaning. The complexity of speech, words, vocabulary and sentence length advance apace thereafter and children gradually become accustomed to the grammar and sounds of their native language. Indeed as their own differentiation becomes more complex they no longer hear certain sounds which are particular to languages other than their own. Intellect plays an increasing part in mature language skills and language is used for the expression of intellectual thought. This is what distinguishes man from animals.

The acquisition of language is a social procedure, i.e. it takes two. Children who have grown up in conditions of extreme deprivation do not develop satisfactory language and it is doubtful whether a child could acquire language from listening to a linguistically varied but unresponsive television set. Language development is divided into and assessed in the following aspects:

Comprehension

How much does the child understand of what is said to him? Children understand before they express and understand more than they can express, as shown by their use of symbolic language. They respond to questions such as 'Where's Daddy?' by looking at him long before they can say 'Daddy'. The close liaison between hearing and understanding of speech is shown by a toddler's ability to call a great many objects on four wheels 'brrm, brrm' before he can say 'car'. Two-year-olds, who called a variety of four-legged animals 'doggies' were, nevertheless, able to point correctly to the dog when shown a picture with several different animals in it (Thompson et al 1977).

Expression

How much can the child say; how complex and correct is his speech and is it appropriate for his age? Assessment of expressive speech is complex. The content of expressive speech is analysed for the ability to use words with meaning and order words in a sentence correctly, i.e. syntactically. Assessment will include executive speech. Speech is not the only form of expression; writing, gesturing and signing are others. Babbling and early sounds have been insufficiently researched. A baby may understand more of his babbling than we imagine as babies can alter the pitch of their babble according to whether they are babbling to their mother or father (Lieberman 1967).

Symbolic or inner language

How well can the child symbolize, i.e. internalize and organize, in order to express verbal material? How good is his coding and intellectualization of language? Give a 15–16-months-old child a full-size hairbrush and he will put it up to his hair making a brushing movement. It may be upside down but never mind! When he is a little older he will brush a doll's hair. He shows comprehension of the word by his action although he certainly cannot yet say 'brush'. Later still, he will be able to play with miniature toys in a similar symbolic manner. The Pollak Making Tea Test (Pollak 1972) makes use of this play with miniatures. A miniature table followed by two chairs are silently handed to a 2- to 3-year-old child. The chairs are automatically put up to the table. If now given two miniature dolls in the seated position, they are placed on the chairs. There are further refinements such as putting the kettle on the cooking stove, making a cup of tea, stirring in the sugar, etc. which allow the test to be used for older children and give a guide to maturity of inner language (Fig. 2.9).

Nonverbal communication

There are two reasons for assessing this part of language development. Firstly, it may be absent or inadequate. Blind and deaf children usually

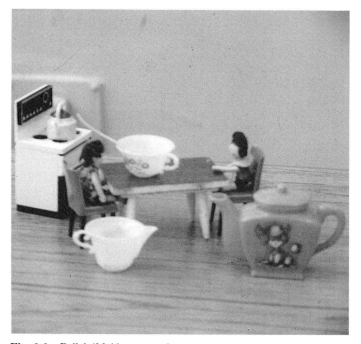

Fig. 2.9 Pollak 'Making tea test'.

have normal facial expressions but aphasic or autistic children do not and the latter lack eye contact. Secondly, nonverbal communication may be present or trainable in children with verbal disorders — this forms the basis of treatment in communication systems such as sign language.

Generally, all linguistic acquisition proceeds through defined phases concurrently. Unless a measure is made of all the above four aspects of communication skills it is not possible to make a diagnosis between language delay and disorder and certainly not a differential diagnosis between linguistic language delay and other causes of verbal delay.

Theories of language development are many and can be divided along the lines of the nature/nurture controversy. The chief of the former is Chomsky (1968, 1975) who suggests the baby has an inborn capacity for language learning. This theory finds support in the fact that there are specific areas of the brain for language and the remarkable amount of language which mentally retarded children are capable of despite their developmental delay. The nurture theorists are those who support the learning theory. Babies and children gradually acquire language from imitation of speech heard and reinforced by adults, a viewpoint helped by the fact that children learn to speak best from teaching adults. The so-called telegraphic speech is not a shortened version of adult speech but a universal child language with its own grammar (Schaffer 1985). In addition to the naturists and empiricists, there is also the interactionist position. Children are biologically prepared to accept language. As the central nervous system develops children are likely to acquire ideas which include linguistic ideas.

There is something to recommend each of these views, but all have inadequacies. The naturist and interactionist views do not take into account the very great influence of environment on language development. In clinical practice it becomes clear that adult language has been acquired by a mixture of many methods so what appears appropriate and helpful can be taken from each of these theories. Although the rate at which language is acquired may differ in different children, all children follow the same rules of word order and go through the same stages of expressing the meaning of words. The development of syntactical rules also follows a pattern. The development of language is, therefore, as amenable to assessment as any other parameter of development and capable of both developmental and differential diagnosis.

Delays in speech and language are extremely common. Due to the environmental influence, it is not surprising that speech delay is much more common in inner city and in lower social class children than those living in the country and in middle class homes. A developmental delay in expressive language has been estimated as occurring in 5–6 per 1000 children (Graham 1986). Children with learning disabilities frequently have a history of late (essentially expressive) language development. A disorder of language development is less common — 1 per 10 000

Beadle M 1970 A child's mind. How children learn during the critical years from birth to age five years. Universal Paperbacks, Methuen, London

Bee H 1981 The developing child. Harper & Row, New York

Bell E T 1937 Men of mathematics. Gollancz, London

Birch H G, Lefford A 1963 Intersensory development in children. Monographs of the Society for Research in Child Development 28

Bower T 1978 The perceptual world of the child. Fontana/Open Books, London

Brown C A 1961 The development of visual capacity in the infant and young child. Cerebral Palsy Bulletin 3: 364

Catford G V, Oliver A 1973 Development of visual acuity. Archives of Disease in Childhood 48: 47–50

Chomsky N 1968 Language and mind. Harcourt Brace Jovanovich, New York

Chomsky N 1975 Reflections on language. Pantheon, New York

DeCasper A J, Fifer W P 1980 Of human bonding: newborns prefer their mothers' voices. Science 208: 1174–1176

Dobbing J, Sands J 1978 Head circumference, biparietal diameter and brain growth in foetal and postnatal life. Early human development 2: 81

Dominick J R, Greenberg B S 1972 Attitudes toward violence: the interaction of television exposure, family attitudes and social class. In: Comstock G A, Rubenstein E A (eds) Television and social behaviour, US Government Printing Office, Washington, vol 3

Douglas J W B, Ross J M, Simpson H R 1967 The ability and attainment of short-sighted pupils. Journal of the Royal Statistical Society 30a: 479

Emes C 1985 Modifying motor behaviour of blind children for participation in sport and physical activity. In: Steadward R (ed) Sport for the disabled. Champian, Human Kinetics Publications, Illinois

Fantz R L 1961 The origin of form perception. Scientific American 204(5): 66

Fantz R L, Fagan J F, Miranda S B 1975 Early visual selectivity. In: Cohen L B, Salapatek P (eds) Infant perception: From sensation to cognition, Academic Press, New York, vol 1

Fraiberg S 1977 Insights from the blind. Comparative studies of blind and sighted infants. Basic Books, New York

Frank P 1948 Einstein, his life and times. Jonathan Cape, London

Frankenburg W K, Dodds J B 1967 The Denver Developmental Screening Test. Journal of Pediatrics 71(2): 181–191

Gardiner P 1969 Refractive errors in relation to physical characteristics and systemic disorders. In: Gardiner P, MacKeith R, Smith V (eds) Aspects of developmental and paediatric ophthalmology. Spastics International, London

Gardner L J 1972 Deprivation dwarfism. Scientific American 227: 76–82

Gardner R A, Gardner B T 1974 Early signs of language in child and chimpanzee. Science 187

Gesell A, Thompson H 1929 Learning and growth in identical twins. Genetic Psychology Monographs 6(1): 1–124

Gibson E J 1969 Principles of perceptual learning and development. Appleton-Century Crofts, New York

Gibson E J, Walk R D 1960 'The visual cliff.' Scientific American 202: 80–92

Graham P 1986 Child psychiatry: a developmental approach. Oxford Medical Publications, Oxford

Griffiths R 1970 The abilities of young children: comprehensive system of mental measurement for the first eight years of life. Test Agency, High Wycombe

Harris D B 1963 Children's drawings as measures of intellectual maturity: a revision and extension of the Goodenough Draw-a-Man Test. Harcourt Brace Jovanovich and World, New York

Holt K S 1979 Development guidance. Child: Care, Health and Development 5: 249–266

Holt K S 1980 Neurological and neuromuscular diseases. In: Gabel S, Erickson M T (eds) Child development and developmental disabilities. Little, Brown and Co, Boston

Holziner K 1939 Student manual of factor analysis. Department of Education, Chicago

Illingworth R S 1987 The developmental history. In: Illingworth R S The development of the infant and young child, 9th edn. Churchill Livingstone, Edinburgh, pp 173–180

King J M, Taitz L S 1985 Catch up growth following abuse. Archives of Disease in Childhood 60: 1152–1154

Liberman I Y, Shankweiler D, Liberman A M, Fowler C, Fischer F W 1976, Phonetic segmentation and recording in the beginning reader. In: Reber A S, Scarborough D (eds) Reading: theory and practice. Erlbaum, Hillsdale, New Jersey

Lieberman P 1967 Interaction, perception and language. MIT Press, Cambridge, Massachusetts

Marinosson G L 1974 Performance profiles of matched normal, educationally subnormal and severely subnormal children on the revised ITPA. Journal of Child Psychology and Psychiatry 15: 139–148

Martin J A M, Moore W J 1979 Childhood deafness in the European community, 111, Commission of the European Communities, EUR 6413

Mathisen B, Skuse D, Wolke D, Reilly S 1989 Oral-motor dysfunction and failure to thrive among inner-city infants. Developmental Medicine/Child Neurology 31: 293–302

McFarlane M 1925 A study of practical ability. British Journal of Psychology Monographs Supplement 8

Nelson M N, Ellen M, Bozynski A et al 1985 Three-year follow-up of >1200g infants: how long should corrected ages be used? Rus-Presbyterian–St Luke's Medical Center, Chicago

Pollak M 1972 Today's three-year-olds in London. Heinemann Medical Books, Oxford

Pollak M 1979 Nine year olds. MTP press, Lancaster

Pollak M, Mitchell S 1974 Early development of negro and white babies. Archives of Disease in Childhood 49: 40–44

Richman N, Stevenson J, Graham P 1982 Pre-school to school: a behavioural study. Academic Press, London

Rodier P M 1980 Chronology of neuron development: animal studies and their clinical implications. Developmental Medicine/Child Neurology 22: 525–545

Rosenblum M F, Finegold D N, Charney E B 1983 Assessment of stature of children with myelomeningocele and usefulness of armspan measurement. Developmental Medicine/Child Neurology 25: 338–342

Rutter M 1980 Introduction. In: Rutter M (ed) Scientific foundations of developmental psychiatry 1. Heinemann Medical Books, Oxford

Rutter M L, Graham P, Chadwick O, Yule W 1976 Adolescent turmoil: fact or fiction? Journal of Child Psychology and Psychiatry 17: 35–56

Rutter M L, Tupling C, Berger M, Yule W 1975 Attainment and adjustment in two geographical areas: 1. Prevalence of psychiatric disorders. British Journal of Psychiatry 126: 493–509

Schlesinger H S, Meadow K P 1972 Sound and sign. University of California Press, Berkeley

Shaffer D R 1985 Developmental psychology, theory, research and applications. Brooks/Cole, Monterey, California

Sheridan M D 1974 What is normal distance vision at five to seven years? Development Medicine/Child Neurology 16: 189–195

Smith I, Macfarlane 1964 Spatial ability: Its educational and social significance. University of London, London

Stayton D, Hogan R, Ainsworth M 1971 Infant obedience and maternal behaviour: origins of socialisation reconsidered. Childhood Development 42: 1057–1069

Stott D H, Moyes F A, Henderson S E 1972 Test of motor impairment. Brook Educational Publications, Ontario

Swineford F 1948 A study in factor-analysis: the nature of the general, verbal and spatial bifactors. Supplementary Educational Monographs 67. University of Chicago Press, Chicago

Tanner J M 1956 Physical and physiological aspects of child development. In: Tanner J M, Inhelder B (eds) Discussions on child development, Tavistock Publications, London, vol 1, p 36

Tanner J M 1978 Foetus into man: physical growth from conception to maturity. Harvard University Press, Cambridge, Massachusetts

Tanner J M, Whitehouse R H, Marshall W A, Healy M J R, Carter B S 1975 Prediction of adult height from height, bone age, and occurrence of menarche at ages 4–16 with allowance for mid-parent height. Archives of Disease in Childhood 50: 14

Tanner J M 1970 Growth and endocrinology of the adolescent. In: Gardner L J (Ed) Endocrine and genetic diseases of childhood. W B Saunders, Philadephia

Thompson J R, Chapman R S 1977 'Who is daddy?' revisited. The status of two-year-olds overextended words in use and comprehension. Journal of Child Language 4: 359–375

Yarrow L J, Rubenstein J I, Pederson F A 1975 Infant and environment. Early cognitive and motivational development. Halsted Press, New York

3. Factors which affect development

There is, at least in the early years, a surprising similarity between the developmental levels of all children around the world (Pollak 1988, Antonovsky et al 1973). On the other hand, as Richman (1972) has pointed out, each individual is different even at birth. Many many factors influence any individual child's development; these might be divided into genetic, environmental, mixed genetic and environmental and pathological.

GENETIC FACTORS

Genetic endowment

Since a human being has approximately 12 000 pairs of chromosomes, the possible combinations of sperm and ovum is of the order of 300 trillion (Lansdown 1984). Genetic endowment is therefore one of the most powerful factors which affect development. It could be said that the effect of the gene (the nucleus) upon the environment (the cytoplasm) is the embryonic blueprint of development. Nor does the influence of genes stop at birth. The case has been made for a lifelong effect (Shields 1980). Some genetically acquired diseases are not present at birth, appearing later, whilst some characteristics appearing in adolescence or adult life, such as addiction and personality disorders, may have a partly genetic basis (Bohman et al 1980, Goodwin et al 1974, 1977). Rutter et al (1963), studying the genetic and environmental effects on 'primary reaction patterns' demonstrated a strong genetic basis for reactions such as activity and approach/withdrawal. Adopted children have been studied to estimate the relative effects of genetic endowment and environment on abnormal behaviour. Analysing the reported literature, Bohman (1981) concluded that genetic factors contribute appreciably to schizophrenia and criminality. The inheritability of intelligence is beyond dispute although estimation of proportions of genetic and environmental factors are not.

Sex

Sex differences are more far-reaching than might be supposed. Growth and motor development are obvious differences but, in the personal/social parameter, boys are more aggressive than girls (Maccoby et Jacklin 1980) whilst girls are more likely to be anxious than boys. It is said that boys have superior visual acuity, making them better shots; girls are earlier in walking and talking. It is not the writer's intention to enter a lion's den by discussing whether there are differences in intellect between the sexes. However, what can be said is that as long as many aspects of society remain 'a man's world' women can expect men to attempt dominance through their greater strength and aggression. This may have the effect that women believe they are intellectually inferior and vice versa! Evidence suggests the female sex is more naturally interested in the care of young children (e.g. Frodi & Lamb 1978) and more emotionally sympathetic towards others (Hoffman 1977).

Sex-linked inheritance of certain congenital malformations is mostly to the disadvantage of males (Winter 1972). The male is at a greater risk both in utero and after birth (Robinson 1969). Males have an increased risk of behavioural disorders, cerebral palsy, epilepsy and mental retardation (Childs 1965). Males are more likely to suffer from hospital admissions, infections, nutritional deficiency and accidents (Winter et Mainzer 1961). The increased resistance of females to infections may be due to differences in the development of immune mechanisms (Childs 1965) and antibody response (Michaels & Rogers 1971).

ENVIRONMENTAL FACTORS

Prenatal influences

The debate about a 'critical' or 'sensitive' period concerns the postnatal period. Evidence suggests there *is* a critical period in prenatal life for normal development of different systems of the fetus and there are examples in experimental embryology when times of maximum sensitivity have been demonstrated (Connolly 1972). Partly, this evidence comes from knowledge of the development of the central nervous system during the prenatal period, partly from the effect of accidents to the central nervous system during critical periods (Rodier (1980) gives an excellent description) and, partly, from the well charted effects of drugs taken during different times of pregnancy. Why only certain drugs affect the *fetus* when a much wider range may affect the *born* child is little understood. A system or organ seems most vulnerable in prenatal life at the time of fastest growth. The period 2–8 weeks after conception is described as the 'fetal sensitive period' because the embryo is particularly sensitive to teratogens during this time (Schaffer 1985). Damage is usually selective. The uterus and the maternal bloodstream almost certainly provide protection from some infections since an organism may affect the child *after* birth yet the fetus seemed unaffected in the *prenatal* period.

Maternal *smoking* in pregnancy is associated with small-for-dates babies

not always possible to continue this family structure and this sometimes causes differences of opinion and conflict between younger and older generations (Lobo 1978). The effect of the average nuclear family upon child development is extremely complex and ill understood. Hinde (1980) has emphasized that the essential ingredients are relationships within the family and the perception of this relationship by both parties. Some major events in family life, or ways in which it can stray from the average nuclear family, e.g. the breakup of the family, the death of a parent or living in a one-parent family, can all affect the child's development. Only some children will be affected and why one child in the family may be affected whilst another remains untouched remains largely a mystery.

Family discord

Marital disharmony affects children's development. Unhappy marriages often cause variability in parental discipline and chaotic household routines. Both are known to affect personalsocial development. Boys appear to be more vulnerable — to all developmental onslaughts — than girls. Antisocial behaviour and delinquency are the more common problems (Jonsson 1967). Behaviour problems in adolescents are more common when children live in discordant rather than happy homes (Rutter et al 1975).

Breakdown of marriage with subsequent separation and divorce

Circumstances which follow family discord are important for development. For example, whether the financial status of the mother and the children deteriorates; if children remain with the mother what relationship is maintained with the father; the age and sex of the children at divorce matters, younger children being more affected than older ones (Wallerstein & Kelly 1975); boys are more vulnerable than girls (Maccoby & Jacklin 1980). Hetherington et al (1978) studied children of both sexes following the divorce of their parents. Both sexes were initially affected. Social relationships with peers and personal low spirits were impaired as was creative play. Both tended towards aggressive behaviour. However one year after the divorce, although play was still stereotyped, girls were much improved and two years afterwards appeared no different to the matched controls. The boys remained more aggressive, less cooperative and more wary of their peers.

Before being confident that no long-term disadvantages ensue, much more research is needed. Children involved in re-marriages and the acquisition of step-siblings who are either (or both) older and younger than themselves need to be studied, particularly their personalsocial development. Depression, difficulties with heterosexual relationships and subsequent difficulties with their own marriages are possible long-term effects (Richards 1982, Fine 1987, Waters & Dimock 1983).

Death of a parent

Childhood bereavement appears to have less effect on children's development than might be supposed. Rutter (1971) found a slight increase in psychiatric disturbance and suggests the long-term effects are greatest when the death occurs when the child is young (Rutter 1972).

One-parent families

The developmental effect of living with one parent is difficult to assess as this is often associated with other factors of disadvantage. Living with one parent with whom the child has a good relationship is better for a child than living with two parents constantly at loggerheads (Rutter 1971). If the one parent has a personality disorder the personalsocial development of the child is likely to be abnormal. I have observed several children, in one-parent homes in which the parent had a psychiatric disorder, who developed severe pseudo-autistic disorders in the sense that when the children came to live in better and happier circumstances 'autism' disappeared and their disordered language gradually improved. Ferri (1976) and Essen (1979), using data from the National Child Development Study (NCDS) when the children were 11 years old and school leavers respectively, expressed the view that the lower school achievements of one-parent children was due to their lower socio-economic status. When background factors were adjusted the apparent lower attainment in reading and mathematics cancelled out. Davie et al (1972) found the reading ages of middle class but not working class children from one-parent homes was lower than those from homes with both parents.

Parents

The parenting of *both* parents affects their child's development. The mixture of genetic and environmental influences upon the developing personality of the child is nowhere better seen than in the effects of parenting, each member of the triad affecting the attitudes of the others which in turn may affect the development of the child. Attitudes of both parents towards the discipline of their children and punishment patterns affects children's moral behaviour (Hoffman 1975). Holmes & Robins (1987) give evidence that unfair, harsh and inconsistent discipline by parents in early years may be associated with later alcoholism and depression. Parental encouragement, intellectual stimulation and creative pursuits were the factors in the home which most highly correlated with general cognitive index and school achievement (Parkinson et al 1982). Swan & Stavros (1973) studying parents of preschool children in a low socio-economic area, discovered that those who encouraged their offspring to have a creative and adventurous attitude towards life; who provided a rich verbal environment and reacted in a non-conflictual way had children with the most effective learning skills.

Certain parental characteristics such as paternal youth, aggression and alcoholism are associated with child abuse. Parents may make one child in the family the scapegoat and this is likely to be the child who is abused. Parents are likely to be experiencing sexual difficulties (White Franklin 1975). Personalsocial and language development are the parameters affected by child abuse. The 'frozen watchfulness' of the battered child is well known (White Franklin 1975). Abused children as young as 2–3 years avoid social contact and lack social skills (George & Main 1979). Children aged 5–10 years who had suffered abuse were abnormally fearful (Jacobson & Straker 1982). Both Sarsfield (1974) and Jacobson & Straker (1982) have noted little study of the children's subsequent development, the major part of published research being concerned with the parents or the abuser rather than the child. In one retrospective study the abused children scored lower on Wechsler Scales of Children's Intelligence (WSCI) and were delayed in language and reading compared with a control group. A twofold increase in psychological problems was noted in adult women who had been sexually abused in childhood (Hooper 1990).

Maternal influences

These are described in more detail in Chapter 8. As the newborn babe lies so often in his mother's arms or is attended by her, their relationship is one of great importance to them both. Whilst the effect of the personality of the mother on the baby is obvious it should be remembered that the baby also has an effect upon the mother (Dunn & Richards 1977). Mothers are affected by the behaviour of older children (Harper 1975). Health visitors who interviewed mothers after delivery and followed up their children's health and development, found severe stresses experienced by the mothers were closely associated with neurological dysfunction, developmental lag and behaviour disturbance in their children (Stott 1973). What happens if this relationship is broken? So much has been written about maternal separation and its effect on behaviour in childhood and later life the reader is referred to Bowlby's (1973) work on the subject which has been briefly described under the ethological theory (Ch. 1) and in Chapter 8. A relationship between maternal depression in a child's first year of life and his later cognitive and language development has been shown (Cox 1988).

In an attempt to study maternal effects separately from the home environment, Pollak (1979) divided the environment of the homes of 200 3-year-olds into the basic fabric and amenities of the home and what stimulation and affection the child was receiving from his mother. The children's development was divided into motor, personalsocial, language and adaptive parameters. Scales of housing and mothering were made and matched against these scales (Tables 3.1 & 3.2). The much greater influence of mothering compared with housing amenities is shown by the fact that only *motor* development was *un*affected by inadequate mothering whilst *no* developmental parameter was affected by inadequate housing.

Table 3.1 Developmental scores of 200 3-year-olds, matched against adequate and inadequate mothering (From Pollak M 1979 Housing and mothering. Archives of Disease in Childhood 54: 54–58, courtesy of the British Medical Association)

Development	Mean Score			p
	Total $(n = 200)$	Inadequate maternal care$(n = 68)$	Adequate maternal care$(n = 132)$	
Motor (Total possible score = 15)	12.92	12.38	13.5	NS
Personal/social (Total possible score = 10)	7.97	6.93	8.80	<0.001
Language development (Total possible score = 14)	7.99	6.64	9.34	<0.001
Adaptive (Total possible score = 12)	7.25	5.67	8.78	<0.001

NS = not significant.

Breast feeding. The influence of breast feeding on development was studied as part of the National Child Development Study (NCDS) and, when intervening social and biological factors were allowed for, vocabulary had a positive correlation (Taylor et al 1984). Whether breast *milk* accounts for this relation can be questioned. This baby, always bottlefed by his mother (Fig 3.1) receives more interpersonal stimulation and social contact than the second bottlefed baby (Fig. 3.2).

Father's role

See also Chapter 8. When a father takes an interest in his child the child's development is enhanced. Personalsocial development is the parameter mostly affected although cognitive and vocabulary development have also been described (Osborn et al 1984). The absence or inadequacy of

Table 3.2 Developmental scores of 200 3-year-olds, matched against adequate and inadequate housing (From Pollak M 1979 Housing and mothering. Archives of Disease in Childhood 54:54–58, courtesy of the British Medical Association)

Development	Mean score			p
	Total ($n = 200$)	Inadequate housing ($n = 89$)	Adequate housing ($n = 11$)	
Motor (Total possible score = 15)	12.92	13.07	12.77	NS
Personal/ Social (Total possible score = 10)	7.85	7.84	7.86	NS
Language (Total possible score = 14)	7.75	7.50	8.0	NS
Adaptive (Total possible score = 12)	7.25	7.2	7.3	NS

NS = not significant.

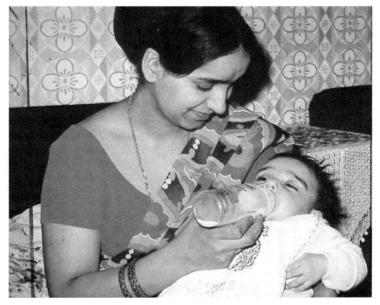

Fig. 3.1 Bottlefed by mother

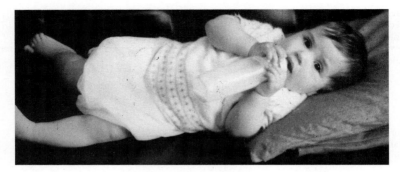

Fig. 3.2   Self-feeding from bottle

fathering correlates significantly with a criminal record by 18–20 years of age (Lewis et al 1982). Despite being an important subject, little has been written of father's attitudes towards their sick and handicapped children. Enwemeka & Andeghe (1982) are exceptions, describing cultural and educational differences in fathers' attitudes towards their handicapped child.

Family size

Children from large families tend towards a lower intelligence quotient and reading age than children from small families (Douglas et al 1968, Stein & Susser 1960, Davie et al 1972, Rutter & Madge 1976, Saunders 1977). The firstborn and the youngest have higher IQs and reading ages than middle children and younger children do better when births are well spaced (Glass et al 1974). The tribulations and advantages of the firstborn have been well described by Fortes (1974).

Siblings

The relationship between siblings is subject to developmental progress; the relationship is likely to be different during a developmental stage of aggression or outgoingness to one of inward reflectiveness (Dunn 1988). Another important factor in sibling relationships is if parents have different attitudes towards individual children perhaps due to the sex and/or temperament of the child (Brody et al 1987).

Twins

Some of the plight of twins are: possible flaws in the estimation of gestational age (James 1980); problems due to the higher risk of abnormal birth

(Gedda 1981); practical problems of having two babies at once leading to problems of bonding (Goshen-Gottstein 1980) and even rejection (Bryan 1983); increased risk of child abuse (Groothius et al 1982); twins scoring lower on IQ tests than non-twins (Silva et al 1982), dizygotic and mono-zygotic twin pairs scoring similarly (Wilson 1981). The 6-month average retardation in the language of 4-year-old twins was considered to be sug-gestive of overall immaturity rather than a linguistic delay (Mittler 1970).

Therefore the main developmental risks for twins are impaired personalsocial development, delayed language and/or lowered IQ when compared with singletons. Despite suggestions to the contrary, twinning has no relation to social class (Murphy & Botting 1989). There is a need for counselling the parents-to-be (Showers 1984). Bryan (1983) provides excellent further reading.

HOME AND HOUSING

Does housing (and/or type) affect children's development? Richman (1974) believes that it does. In her follow-up of mothers and young babies living in high-rise and low-rise (less than four floors) flats and houses, she found that although there was no difference between the three groups in behaviour problems in the children or psychiatric disturbance in the mothers, more mothers in the two former types of housing were depressed and lonely. Both these conditions in mothers are known to affect personalsocial development in children. A report from Shelter (Furley 1989) shows that poor housing, apart from affecting children's health, is associated with poor school performance and affects emotional development. Crowded and poor homes were associated with low reading and mathematic scores in children 16 years old (NCDS) (Essen et al 1978), confirming findings when the children were 7 (Davie et al 1972) and 11 years old (Fogelman 1975). Much has been written about home environment and poor scholastic skills but rarely have the characteristics of the home or housing been studied, the facilities of the housing being combined with financial aspects, childrearing practices and stimulation practices (Dunst & Leet 1987). When the Family Resource Scale (Parkinson et al 1982) tried to tease out from the home environment which factors correlated with the general cognitive index and school progress of children the fabric and amenities of the children's housing were not mentioned. The amenities of the home and the effects of parental care were separated in the study of Pollak (1979). None of the four developmental parameters measured was affected by the adequacy or inadequacy of the amenities or overcrowding of the home. Living in high-rise flats and lack of play facilities have been associated with aggressive behaviour and poor social development in the children (Table 3.2) (Chiltern 1985, Nilsson 1985). If the housing of normal children has been little studied, even less so has the housing of ESN children. Saunders

(1977) is a notable exception. The homes of the ESN(M) children were not any more overcrowded than the mean occupancy rate for Bradford as a whole.

SCHOOL

In the 1960s, Douglas et al (1968), in pioneering studies, demonstrated that intelligence and family lifestyle were the most important factors in school achievement. The Plowden Report (1967) strongly reinforced these findings. As a result there arose an assumption that schools, their teachers and the classroom mattered little. However, in 1972, Power et al (1972) studied juvenile delinquency rates in a London borough and made the interesting observation that the majority of delinquents were pupils from a small number of the schools. Most schools had low rates of delinquency — a finding confirmed by others. It became pertinent, therefore, to consider what was different about these schools. In *Fifteen Thousand Hours*, Rutter et al (1979) studied schools in an inner London borough. Schools were found to make a difference to both children's behaviour and achievement. Some schools consistently produced good results, whilst others within the same catchment area, had consistently bad results in school attainments, pupil behaviour and truancy rates. Factors such as teacher motivation have been shown, in Japanese schools, to help high academic success rate and the pupils' motivation (Cummings 1980, Passow et al 1976).

CULTURE AND SOCIAL CLASS

Culture

What is culture? A fine definition was made by Tylor (1889): that complex whole which includes knowledge, belief, art, law, custom and other capabilities and habits acquired by man as a member of society. Although the prevailing view (e.g. Quinton 1980, Lester 1967, Tizard & Rees 1974) appears to be that cross-cultural studies have too many variables to render any developmental differences found meaningful, there are well made research studies which suggest differing cultural childrearing practices resulted in different developmental trends. For example, Mintern & Lambert (1964) described mothers in six cultures. Comparing Indians in Mexico with Africans in Nyansongo they demonstrated fairly conclusively that differences in parental attitudes and childrearing practices produced different types of behaviour in their children. It is accepted that parental care, including discipline and punishment and different family values, can affect a child's personalsocial development. It does not therefore seem too far-fetched to believe that childrearing practices which differ due to cultural mores may have differing effects. Brazelton (1973) has described how the passivity and lack of aggression of Mayan Indian mothers produced a newborn babe who was quiet yet neurologically advanced. The experience of living in an extended family may be different to growing up in a nuclear one. For example, social skills in the former may have to develop at an earlier age and Mitchell's (1971) study of housing in Hong Kong is interesting in this respect. It was discovered that the very high level of overcrowding was only tolerated when the other multi-occupants were relatives and totally intolerable if the occupants were strangers. (Unfortunately, nothing of the development of the children is noted.)

In some circles (e.g. Plewis 1981, Tizard & Plewis 1977) there has been the view that any cultural or ethnic differences in the development of children of different races was not a permissible subject for discussion but this viewpoint has almost certainly been superseded. There are several respectable studies in which differences have been found. For example, the early advanced motor development of negro babies has been noted by Scott (1975) in West Indian babies in London; Pollak & Mitchell (1974) studying West Indian babies in London; Geber et al (1964) assessing Ugandan babies in Uganda and Super (1976) testing Kenyan babies in Kenya. The latter thought this early advanced development was the result of cultural differences in early motor stimulation. All studies concerned babies in the first years of life and generally, the precocity had disappeared by the second year of life. However, a study of 162 Yoruba school children used the absence of associated movements as a reflection of advanced motor maturity and found their motor development was more mature than Caucasian norms (Ashton 1973). Japanese babies in Tokyo were later in holding up their heads, rolling over and, at an older age, in some aspects of language development compared with Denver (Bryant et al 1974) norms (Ueda 1978). The authors ascribe these differences to differing cultural childrearing practices.

Different cultural childrearing practices were used to explain differences between the three socio-cultural groups in Yucatan, Mexico and Bayley norms. Although the groups did not differ between themselves, their fine motor-coordination was in advance and they were delayed in walking (Solomons & Solomons 1975). Epir & Yalaz (1984) report cultural differences of fine-motor development and linguistic skills in urban Turkish children which could not be accounted for by social class differences.

Three-year-olds from 15 ethnic groups in different areas of the world showed remarkable similarity in development (Pollak 1988). But three groups showed differences in some developmental parameters. The personalsocial development of the Ethiopean refugees in Israel lagged behind that of the others. The Ethiopean children had suffered great privation and transitory lifestyles until they reached Israel. The children of West Indian immigrants in London and 3-year-old American negros in South Carolina were lower in language and nonverbal skills. The two latter groups were disadvantaged in having much less of their mother's time and attention, day by day, than any of the 13 other groups and the London-born West Indians suffered from poorer housing compared with London-born English children. Both the West Indian and American negro children were disadvantaged in more frequently living in one-parent families, in having no regular male figure at home but sharing home with stepsiblings.

Social class

Social class is usually measured in the UK by the registrar-general's classification of occupation of head of the household (although there are well known problems with this classification it is still widely used and serves its purpose provided the disadvantages are known). Social class is an important variable in children's development. Being a member of the *lower social class* (i.e. the unskilled and the unemployed) is associated with a variety of developmental problems including:

Lower intelligence. In a study in five European capitals — London, Paris, Zurich, Stockholm and Brussels — preschool children were examined at ages 1, 3 and 5 years (Graffar & Corbier 1972). In all centres, poor socio-economic class correlated with poor height and weight at age 1 year. This disadvantage remained at 3 and 5 years but was less and no differences in bone maturation were found. For mental development, on the other hand, exactly the opposite was true. No social class differences in mental attainment were found at 1 year but clear differences at 3 and more marked differences at 5 years. The Terman-Merrill test was used and the distinguished authors conclude 'the influence of social factors on the mental development remains considerable and becomes more important with age'. Since this large international study similar conclusions have been reached in many other studies (e.g. Plowden 1967, Douglas et al 1968, Davie et al 1972).

Delayed language development. In a large survey of babies in Nottingham, it was found that lower social class children attained low language levels (Newsom & Newsom 1963, 1968). Bernstein (1965) defined social class differences in language development and suggested how lower social class children's language might disadvantage them especially when they go to school. These findings have been subject to criticism but even a casual observation will note that middle-class language has both explanations and intellectual content that allow it to be a learning tool for a child, which is not so evident in lower-class language. In a Swiss study the effects of pre-, peri- and postnatal events on developmental outcome at 5–7 years of age were studied (Largo et al 1989). The conclusion was that socio-economic status rather than perinatal variables and weight was strongly related to language and intellectual development.

Poor school achievement. The reasons for lower school achievement of lower social class children are multifactorial but their occurrence has been amply demonstrated in the National Child Development Study

(Davie et al 1972) and others. Lower reading ages and specific reading retardation are more common in children of lower social classes (Rutter et al 1970, Jencks et al 1973). Approximately one child in 5 in the Inner London Educational Authority (with a predominance of lower social class pupils) has a reading age at least two years below chronological age. The NCDS (Douglas & Ross 1964) discovered a social class difference between achievement of verbal and mathematical skills and physical maturity. Lower social class boys who matured early were superior in performance to late maturers — a finding which did not apply to middle-class boys. This intriguing observation has been confirmed by Westin-Lindgren (1982).

   Delinquency. A relationship between delinquency and lower social class exists (Quinton 1980) although the association with social class is not well established because it has proved difficult to unravel this influence from other deprivational factors with which lower social class is so often associated.

POVERTY AND THE CYCLE OF DEPRIVATION

Poverty as a problem may be seen as only affecting the underdeveloped countries. This is far from the case. Poverty in all countries of the world has effects on child development. In Britain in 1985 nearly one-fifth of children were living in poverty (Child Poverty Action Group 1988). Hansen (1979) has described povertystricken areas of the USA. Mothers living in poverty are likely to be poorly nourished. For example, in the UK a single woman aged 24 years and expecting her first baby would have to spend 54% of her income to eat the recommended antenatal diet (*British Medical Journal* 1989). She is likely to give birth to a low birthweight and premature baby (Shelter 1988). She and her baby are likely to live in poor housing and lead poorly organized lives (Furley 1989). All these factors will affect her baby's development. Parents living in poverty are less likely to seek available services, with further detriment to the children's development (Phillips et al 1986, Wise et al 1985). Apart from health hazards, these results of poverty are associated with child abuse, delinquency, truancy, poor school achievement, learning disorders and poor language development. Children living in poverty fare less well in all these important developmental parameters (Rutter & Madge 1981, Herbert & Wilson 1977). Later in life, medical conditions such as ischaemic heart disease, stroke, chronic bronchitis and emphysema have all been related to poor maternal health, poor infant feeding and housing conditions (Barker 1988).

The cycle of deprivation

To tease out the individual contribution which social class, poverty, poor housing and/or disorganized lifestyle make to a less than optimum development is difficult. All these factors are usually enmeshed in an inextricable fashion. The phrase 'cycle of deprivation' has been coined and describes the position well and the cycle has never been better described than in the Black Report (1980). One has only to read the biennial 'Social Trends' (HMSO) or the annual 'State of the World's Children' (UNICEF) to note large areas of the world are becoming poorer each year with children the main sufferers, being subject to developmental disadvantages. Yet, however difficult it may be to bring up a family in bed-and-breakfast hotels, in slums and on the poverty line, some parents are able to do this successfully. One can but admire their fortitude and it is an extremely interesting question to ask what are the factors which seem to lead to success? Time and again, the *quality* of family life, the warmth, the love and continued care and concern are the factors most likely to allow a growing child to develop harmoniously and venture out and explore his environment successfully. This view receives support from the study of Cornia (1984) in which there was a successful transformation of family health in Sri Lanka following an educational programme for girls and women. The poverty line remained unchanged (WHO 1984). Swan & Stavros (1973), studying low socio-economic groups in the USA, demonstrated that those children whose parents interacted frequently by encouragement and help were the children verbally and cognitively in advance of children in similar economic conditions but whose parents did not have the same philosophies towards them. Neligan & Prudham (1976), using information from the Newcastle survey on child development, concluded the most important factor affecting the children's development was the quality of the mother's care of her child in the first three years of life.

It is generally supposed that the breaking of the cycle of deprivation is largely financial; this may well be true but these last studies suggest this is not entirely the case.

MIXED GENETIC AND ENVIRONMENT FACTORS

Intelligence

Genetic endowment is needed for the possibility of mental skills and a subtle intermix with environmental influences will bring this potential to full maturity. Argument about the ratio of genetic endowment to environment in the development of intelligence can be left to others.

Temperament

Different types of temperament are described in Chapter 8. Personalsocial development is most affected but since temperament also concerns concentration, attention span and emotional development can be affected in this way. It has been suggested that difficult babies often have hyperanxious mothers although whether this is genetically based or environmental is not clear (Sameroff et al 1975). Characteristics of temperament tend to remain constant but can be modified by family and other environmental dynamics during the child's growth to maturity. It is therefore impossible to be dogmatic about the role that temperament plays in affecting development, since the reverse is also true, i.e. development can affect temperament.

PATHOLOGICAL FACTORS

The developing brain is at risk from many hazards which may cause developmental delays, retardation and abnormalities. Many medical conditions, congenital or acquired, will affect a child's development. Babies who are classified as 'neurologically suspect' will consistently perform below control children on measures of intelligence, language development, motor skills and school achievement even when social class and birthweight are controlled (e.g. Rubin & Barlow 1980). On the other hand one can also be more positive and state that if a baby has a normal developmental status between 16–52 weeks of age, the likelihood of having a school-age IQ less than 75 is: 5% if the neuromotor status was normal; 25% if there were minor neurological abnormalities; 45% if there were major neurological abnormalities (Knobloch et al 1974).

Amongst *congenital* causes, inherited metabolic inborn errors of metabolism and chromosomal abnormalities are the most important. Drugs taken in pregnancy and maternal infections such as toxoplasmosis and AIDS (Ultmann et al 1985) have to be considered in *prenatal* causes. Another hazard is the interference of aminoacid and protein synthesis as in, for example, phenylketonuria.

Perinatal causes are birth injury and brain and neonatal convulsions. Imbalance of hormones and biochemistry and malnutrition all affect development since function of the central nervous system is affected. Low brainweight and lowered postnatal cell formation are the two most common results. The plight of the low-birthweight baby has already been described but Davis (1970) reminds that these babies are smaller and less intelligent than controls right up to adult life. In another study of high-risk premature and mature infants with *fetal-newborn complications* cognitive and motor deficits were found in 24% at age 1 year, 14% having one or more major, and 10% one or more minor, deficits. These deficits have been found to have an association with fetal hypoxia, newborn respiratory complications and newborn encephalopathy (Low et al 1985).

Some of the more important *postnatal medical* causes are:

Epilepsy. Gowers (1907), one of the pioneers of modern views on epilepsy, first reported that most patients with epilepsy were of normal mental intelligence and serious psychiatric and behavioural problems were usually consequent upon having a pathological lesion of the brain. However, epilepsy is often associated with developmental problems. Neonatal convulsions and infantile spasms (the aetiology of which is varied) are often associated with underlying brain disease and thus with mental retardation (Illingworth 1987). An age of under 1 year for the onset of infantile febrile status epilepticus carries a grave prognosis (Viani et al 1987). Epilepsy of late onset, particularly petit mal, is associated with learning problems, mostly of the visuospatial type (Stores 1971, 1978). Behaviour problems are common (Lindsey et al 1979) and have been shown to be related to damage of the central nervous system (Hoare 1984). Despite the effects of anticonvulsants and the seizures themselves, linear length has not been shown to be affected (Tada et al 1986). Smith & Wallace (1982) followed up children after discharge from hospital after their first *febrile convulsion*. Children who suffered a further fit showed a decrease on the Griffiths scales, whereas children who suffered no further fits showed an increase. It was suggested that the risk to intellectual function of a further fit is higher than the risk of continuous medication.

Head injury. Learning and behavioural changes are reported after severe head injuries (Shaffer 1973, Chadwick et al 1981).

Neoplasms and irradiation. Cause and effect are difficult to separate but learning and behavioural deficits have been reported after both. The younger the child the greater is the effect. Children with treated solid tumours were not found to be different to normal children on scores for IQ, reading, memory and learning. Children with lymphoblastic leukaemia treated with irradiation and chemotherapy had lower scores on all these tasks. This was most marked when the children were under 5 years of age (Eiser 1980). Children with treated solid tumours were lower intellectually but children with acute lymphoblastic leukaemia even more so in the study by Twaddle et al (1983) but when followed up two years later the deficits in intellectual functioning had not deteriorated (Twaddle et al 1986). In another study, children with lymphoblastic leukaemia in remission after treatment were compared with their siblings on standardized IQ and attainment tests. Although within average range, all the leukaemic children were lower than their siblings except those who had treatment after 7 years of age. Those treated under 3 years of age were markedly lower (Jannoun 1983).

Infections (especially meningitis). Less than 10% of children suffer sequelae after meningitis. When they do it is usually a lowering of IQ and learning problems which ensue. The younger the child the more likely the damage.

Malnutrition. In a westernized country it is difficult to realize that approximately 100 million children in the world suffer from malnutrition. The greatest developmental effect of poor food intake is stunting of physical and cerebral growth. Three groups of Ugandan children all of whom had suffered protein-energy malnutrition in early childhood were compared with carefully matched controls. The malnourished children, aged between 11 and 17 years, were significantly below the controls in anthropometric measurements and tests of intellectual ability. Reasoning and spatial abilities were most affected; memory and rote learning intermediate whilst language was scarcely affected at all (Hoorweg et al 1976). Cravioto & Robles (1965) and Madge & Tizard (1980) both mention attention deficits and learning problems as sequelae of malnutrition. A mother's dietary state is likely to affect the dietary state of her child (Ojofeitimi 1984). Whether physical and mental stunting is permanent is less certain.

Korean girls, all of whom had been malnourished, were adopted into middle-class American homes and their heights, weights and IQs all improved and caught up with Korean averages (Lansdown 1984). Children whose nutritional status improves sometimes show rapid improvements in developmental lags (Cravioto & Robles 1965, Yatkin & McLaren 1970) although the rises in developmental quotients have been attributed to improvements in happiness and health rather than overcoming the results of malnutrition (Grantham-McGregor et al 1978).

Severe *mal*nutrition which largely affects children in underdeveloped countries has to be distinguished from *under*nutrition which is more common in developed countries. There is no consensus of the end results of undernutrition. These children often suffer from the cycle of deprivation so it is not clear what effect undernutrition plays in their later development (Lloyd-Still 1976, Stein et al 1976). Dobbing (1987) gives an excellent review of many factors involved and Holt (1982) an account of the relationship between development and nutritional factors. Lucas et al (1989) suggest that low birthweight babies who are fed on preterm formula rather than donor breast milk will have superior developmental quotients at 9 months. The message would seem to be that whilst sending grain can help to fight malnutrition, the follow-up with an adequate lifestyle and intellectual stimulation is also necessary.

Iron deficiency anaemia. There are reports that iron defiency can cause lack of concentration (Howell 1971), and impaired developmental scores (Tucker et al 1981). Changes are small but iron deficiency is common because of delayed weaning, artificial feeding and maternal anaemia in pregnancy (Illingworth 1986). Diagnosing and treating is worthwhile because a marked improvement in concentration span may follow (Evans 1985). This improvement has not been noted in other anaemias. Evans suggests iron is involved with metabolic pathways leading to changes in cell function which accounts for the improvements. Similar improvements were reported by Aukett et al (1986).

Hypothyroidism. Treating congenital hypothyroidism gives encouraging results. Murphy et al (1986), reporting on the follow-up at 1, 3 and 5 years of babies discovered by neonatal screening and treated, found developmental scores within the normal range with the exception of motor skills. A study in northern England (Birrell et al 1983) found no significant differences in IQ to controls but the treated hypothyroid children were less coordinated and had more behavioural problems. These authors believe treatment must be instigated within one month of birth. An earlier study from Russia (Skorodok 1969) had clearly demonstrated the crucial role that early diagnosis plays in prognosis.

Lead. Overt lead poisoning is rare in the UK but the diagnosis is usually clear. Lead paint, putty, surma (an eye cosmetic) and a baby tonic (the two latter are seen amongst Asians) are the most common sources of lead. Lead poisoning has been associated with reduced IQs and learning skills. Until the study of Yule et al (1981) blood lead concentrations below 35 ug/100 ml were not considered to have deleterious effects on children. However, this study assessed children with blood lead levels of 7–33 mg/100 ml on a battery of psychometric tests. Significant associations between blood lead levels and reading and spelling ability and IQ, but not mathematics, were obtained which remained even when social class was taken into account. These results question the significance of lead levels below those of toxicity but above those considered normal.

Several studies (McNeil & Plasnik 1974 in Texas; Lansdown et al 1974 in London; Hebel et al 1976 in Birmingham) failed to find lower IQ or learning skills in children all of whom were living in areas exposed to lead pollution whilst in a recent study in Italy (Bergomi et al 1989) results on WSCI were affected by levels of lead which were within the ranges observed in urban areas. This debate continues. It has been argued that higher lead levels are likely to be associated with lower socio-economic status, itself associated with lower reading, spelling and IQ (Bax 1981). Several studies demonstrate improvement in intellectual and behavioural function after treatment (e.g. David 1978, David et al 1976). Even in 1964 Montcrieff et al were drawing attention to the frequent finding of raised blood lead levels in children with mental handicap, severe behaviour disorder and pica and the majority of these blood lead levels did not reach poisoning levels (BMJ 1977). Readers who are interested are recommended to read the excellent book by Lansdown et al (1986).

Solvent abuse. There is evidence that chronic solvent abuse, by carrying an increased risk of cognitive impairment and depression, has implications for verbal, nonverbal and personalsocial development (Zur et al 1990).

Conclusion

This chapter has described the major factors that may affect a child's development. The factors have been presented separately but, in reality, a child's development is multifactorial. Of the many studies that attempt to distinguish the relative importance of different factors affecting a child's development the prospective 9-year follow-up study of Lindahl et al (1988) is one of the most comprehensive. The most significant predictors of neurodevelopmental problems at age 9 which this study showed were :

1. Smallness for gestational age
2. Neonatal signs of cerebral depression
3. Low social class.

How better could the intertwining of prenatal, natal and postnatal factors be demonstrated? It might seem that no two children can possibly develop in the same way; it can only be reiterated that if the miracle of life is that every child is *different* it is even more magical that every child is so *similar*.

REFERENCES

Alberman E, Benson J, McDonald A 1982 Cerebral palsy and severe educational subnormality in low-birthweight children: a comparison of births in 1951–53 and 1970–73. Lancet i: 606–8

Antonovsky H F, Feitelson D 1973 An observational study of intellectual stimulation of young children. Early Child Development and Care 2: 329–344

Ashton R 1973 Associated movements in Yoruba school children. Developmental Medicine and Child Neurology 15: 3–7

Astbury J, Orgill A, Bajuk B 1987 Relationship between two year behaviour and neurodevelopmental outcome at five years if very low birthweight survivors. Developmental Medicine and Child Neurology 29: 370–379

Astbury J, Orgill A A, Bajuk B, Yu V Y H 1983 Determinants of developmental performance of very low birthweight survivors at one and two years of age. Developmental Medicine and Child Neurology 25: 709–716

Aukett M A, Parks Y A, Scott P H, Wharton B A 1986 Treatment with iron increases weight gain and psychomotor development. Archives of Disease in Childhood 61: 849–857

Barker D J P 1988 Childhood causes of adult diseases. Archives of Disease in Childhood 63: 867–869

Bax M 1981 Lead and impaired abilities. Developmental Medicine and Child Neurology 23: 565–566

Bergomi M, Borella P, Fantuzzi G et al 1989 Relationship between lead exposure indicators and neuropsychological performance in children. Developmental Medicine and Child Neurology 31: 181–190

Bernstein B 1965 A socio-linguistic approach to social learning. In: Gould C (ed) Survey of the social sciences. Penguin, Harmondsworth

Bill J M, Sykes D H, Hoy E A 1986 Difficulties in comparing outcomes of low-birthweight studies because of obsolescent test norms. Developmental Medicine and Child Neurology 28: 244–250

Birrell J, Frost G J, Parkin J M 1983 The development of children with congenital hypothyroidism. Developmental Medicine and Child Neurology 25: 512–519

Bohman M 1981 The interaction of heredity and childhood environment: some adoption studies. Journal of Child Psychology and Psychiatry 22: 195–200

Bohman M, Sigvarsson S 1980 A prospective, longitudinal study of children registered for adoption: a 15 year follow-up. Acta Psychiatrica Scandinavica 61: 339–355

Bowlby J 1951 Maternal care and mental health. HMSO, London

Bowlby J 1958 The nature of the child's tie to his mother. International Journal of Psychoanalysis 39: 350

Bowlby J 1969 Attachment and loss, vol 1. Hogarth Press, London

Bowlby J 1973 Attachment and loss, Hogarth Press, London, vol 2.

Brazelton T B 1973 Effect of maternal expectations on early infant behaviour. Early Child Development and Care 2: 259–273

British Medical Journal 1981 Editorial. Helping the child at risk. 282: 1647–1648
British Medical Journal 1977 Child Health and environmental lead : 255–256
British Medical Journal 1989 In Britain: not the decade of the child 298: 8
Brody G H, Stoneman Z, Burke M 1987 Child temperaments, maternal differential behavior and sibling relationships. Development Psychology 23: 354–362
Brown J K, Purvis R J, Forfar J O, Cockburn F 1974 Neurological aspects of perinatal asphyxia. Developmental Medicine and Child Neurology 16: 567–580
Bryan E M 1983 The nature and nurture of twins. Baillière Tindall, London
Bryant G M, Davies K J, Newcombe R G 1974 The Denver developmental screening test. Achievement of test items in the first year of life by Denver and Cardiff infants. Developmental Medicine and Child Neurology 16: 475–484
Butler N R, Goldstein H 1973 Smoking in pregnancy and subsequent child development. British Medical Journal 4: 573–575
Chadwick O, Rutter M, Thompson J, Shaffer D 1981 Intellectual performance and reading skills after localised head injury in childhood. Journal of Child Psychology and Psychiatry and Allied Disciplines 22: 117
Chandler L S, Andrews M S, Swanson M W 1980 The movement assessment of infants. A manual. Rolling Bay, Washington
Child Poverty Action Group 1988. Poverty, the facts
Childs B 1965 Genetic origin of some sex differences among human beings. Pediatrics 35: 798
Chiltern T 1985 Making the city fit the child.
Clarke A D B 1972 Consistency and variability in the growth of human characteristics. Developmental Medicine and Child Neurology 14: 668–683
Clarke A M, Clarke A D B 1976 Early experience: myth and evidence. Open Books, London
Connolly K 1972 Learning and the concept of critical periods in infancy. Developmental Medicine and Child Neurology 14: 705–714
Cooke R W I, Davies P A 1988 The care of new-born babies — some developments and dilemmas. In: Forfar J O (ed) Child health in a changing society. Oxford University Press
Cornia G A 1984 A summary and interpretation of the evidence. In: Jolly R, Cornia G A (eds) The impact of the world recession on children. Pergamon Press, Oxford
Cox A D 1988 Maternal depression and impact on children's development. Archives of Disease in Childhood 63: 90–95
Cravioto J, Robles B 1965 Evaluation of adaptive and motor behaviour during rehabilitation from Kwashiorkor. American Journal of Orthopsychiatry 35: 449
Cummings W K (1980) Education and equality in Japan. Princeton University Press, Princeton
David O J 1978 Sub-clinical effects of lead on children. Proceedings of Conference on Lead pollution: Health Effects. Conservation Society, London
David O J, Hoffman S, Sverd J, Clark J, Voeller K 1976 Lead and hyperactivity – behavioural response to chelation: a pilot study. American Journal of Psychiatry 133: 1155–1158
Davie R, Butler N, Goldstein H 1972 From birth to seven: a report on the National Child Development Study. Longman, London
Davies P A 1989 More on follow-up studies of low-birthweight infants. Editorial. Developmental Medicine and Child Neurology 31: 143–144
Davis J 1970 The effects of early development on later development. Developmental Medicine and Child Neurology 12: 98–107
Dobbing J 1987 Early nutrition and later achievement. Academic Press, London
Douglas J W R, Ross J M, Simpson H R 1968 All our future: a longitudinal study of secondary education. Davies, London
Douglas J V B, Ross J M 1964 Age of puberty related to educational ability, attainment and school leaving age. Journal of Child Psychology and Psychiatry and Allied Disciplines 5: 185–196
Douglas J W B 1969 Effects of early environment on later development. Journal of the Royal College of Physicians 3: 359
Douglas J W B 1975 Early hospital admissions and later disturbances of behaviour and learning. Developmental Medicine and Child Neurology 17: 294–302
Drillien C M 1964 The growth and development of the prematurely born infant. E & S Livingstone, Edinburgh

Dunn H G 1986 Sequelae of low birthweight: the Vancouver Study. Clinics in Developmental Medicine 95/96. Blackwells, Oxford

Dunn H G, Grunau R V E McBurney A K, McCormick A Q, Schulzer M 1980 Neurological, psychological and educational sequelae of low birthweight. Brain and Development 2: 57–67

Dunn J 1988 Sibling influences on childhood development. Annotation. Journal of Child Psychology and Psychiatry 29.2: 119–127

Dunn J B, Richards M P M 1977 Observations on the developing relationship between mother and baby in the neonatal period. In: Schaffer H R (ed) Studies in mother–infant interaction. Academic Press, London

Dunst C J, Leet H E 1987 Measuring the adequacy of resources in households with young children. Child: Care, Health and Development 13: 111–125

Eiser C 1980 Effects of chronic illness on intellectual development: a comparison of normal children with those treated for childhood leukaemia and solid tumours. Archives of Disease in Childhood 55: 766–771

Elliman A M, Bryan E, Elliman A D 1986 Low birth weight babies at 3 years of age. Child: Care, Health and Development 12: 287–311

Enwemeka C S, Adeghe N U 1982 Some family problems associated with the presence of a child with handicap in Nigeria. Child: Care, Health and Development 8: 133–141

Epir S, Yalaz K 1984 Urban Turkish children's performance on the Denver developmental screening test. Developmental Medicine and Child Neurology 26: 632–643

Eskenazi B, Gaylord L, Bracken M B, Brown D 1988 In utero exposure to organic solvents and human neurodevelopment. Developmental Medicine and Child Neurology 30: 492–501

Essen J 1979 Living in one-parent families: attainment at school. Child: Care, Health and Development 5: 189–200

Essen J, Fogelman K, Head J 1978 Childhood housing experiences and school attainment. Child: Care, Health and Development 4: 41–58

Evans D I K 1985 Cerebral function in iron deficiency: a review. Child: Care, Health and Development 11: 105–112

Ferrari F, Grosoli M V, Fontana G, Cavazuti G B 1980 Neurobehavioural comparison of low risk preterm and fullterm infants at term conceptional age. Developmental Medicine and Child Neurology 25: 450–458

Ferri E 1976 Growing up in a one-parent family: a long term study of child development. National Foundation for Educational Research, Slough

Ferry P C 1981 On growing new neurons: are early intervention programs effective? Pediatrics 67: 38–41

Fine S 1987 Children in divorce, custody and access situations: an update. Annotation. Journal of Child Psychology and Psychiatry and Allied Disciplines 28.3: 361–364

Fogelman K R 1975 Developmental correlates of family size. British Journal of Social Work 5: 43–57

Folio R, Dubose R F 1974 Peabody Motor Scales. Peabody College, Tennessee

Fortes M 1974 The first born. Journal of Child Psychology and Psychiatry and Allied Disciplines 15: 81–104

Frodi A, Lamb M 1978 Sex differences in responsiveness to infants: a developmental study of psychophysical and behavioral responses. Child Development 49: 1182–1188

Furley A 1989 A bad start in life – children, health and housing. Shelter, 88 Old St, London

Geber M, Dean R F 1957 Gesell tests on African children. Pediatrics 20: 1055

Geber M, Dean R F 1964 Le developpment psychomoteur et somatique des jeunes enfants Africains en Ouganda. Courrier 14: 425

Gedda L 1981 The human twin. Progress in Clinical and Biological Research 69b: 1–7

George C, Main M 1979 Social interactions of young abused children: approach, avoidance and aggression. Child Development 50: 306–318

Glass D C, Neulinger J, Brim O G 1974 Birth order, verbal intelligence and educational aspirations. Child Development 45: 807

Goodwin D W, Schulsinger F, Knop J, Mednick S, Guze S 1977 Alcoholism and depression in adopted-out daughters of alcoholics. Archives of General Psychiatry 35: 751–755

Goodwin D W, Schulsinger F, Mollier N, Hermansen L, Winokur G, Guze S B 1974 Drinking problems in adopted and nonadopted sons of alcoholics. Archives of General Psychiatry 31: 164–169

Goshen-Gottstein E R 1980 Mothering of twins, triplets and quadruplets. Psychiatry 43: 189–204

Gowers W 1907 The borderlands of epilepsy.

Graffar M, Corbier J 1972 Contribution to the study of the influence of socio-economic conditions on the growth and development of the child. Early Child Development and Care 1: 141–179

Grantham-McGregor S M, Stewart M, Desai P 1978 A new look at the assessment of mental development in young children recovering from severe malnutrition. Developmental Medicine and Child Neurology 20: 773–778

Griffiths R 1954 The abilities of babies. A study in mental measurement. University of London Press, London

Groothius J R, Altemeier W A, Robarge J P et al 1982 Increased child abuse in families with twins. Pediatrics 70: 769–773

Hansen C M 1979 Child health problems and programmes in two underdeveloped areas of the USA. Child: Care, Health and Development 5: 323–334

Harper L V 1975 The scope of offspring effects: from caregiver to culture. Psychological Bulletin 82: 784–801

Harris S R 1987 Early neuromotor predictors of cerebral palsy in low-birthweight infants. Developmental Medicine and Child Neurology 29: 508–519

Hebel J R, Kinch D, Armstrong E 1976 British Journal of Preventive and Social Medicine 30: 170

Herbert G W, Wilson H 1977 Socially handicapped children. Child: Care, Health and Development 3: 13–21

Hess E H 1959 Imprinting: an effect of early experience. Science 130: 133–141

Hetherington E M, Cox M, Cox R 1981 Play and social interaction in children following divorce. Journal of Social Issues

Hinde R 1980 Family influences. In: Rutter M (ed) Scientific foundations of developmental psychiatry. Heinemann Medical Books, London

Hinde R A 1970 Animal behaviour. A synthesis of ethology and comparative psychology. McGraw-Hill, New York

Hoare P 1984 The development of psychiatric disorder among schoolchildren with epilepsy. Developmental Medicine and Child Neurology 26.3: 3–13

Hoffman M L 1977 Sex differences in empathy and related behaviors. Psychology Bulletin 84: 712–722

Holmes S J, Robins L N 1987 The influence of childhood disciplinary experience on the development of alcoholism and depression. Journal of Child Psychology and Psychiatry and Allied Disciplines 28.3: 399–415

Holt K S 1982 Diets and development. Child: Care, Health and Development 8: 183–201

Hooper P D 1990 Psychological sequelae of sexual abuse in childhood. British Journal of General Practice 40: 29–31

Hoorweg J, Stanfield J P 1976 The effects of protein energy malnutrition in early childhood on intellectual and motor abilities in later childhood and adolescence. Developmental Medicine and Child Neurology 18: 33–350

Horwood S P, Boyle M H, Torrance G W, Sinclair J C 1982 Mortality and morbidity of 500- to 1499-gram birthweight infants live-born to residents of a defined geographic region before and after neonatal intensive care. Pediatrics 69: 613–20

Howell D 1971 Significance of iron deficiencies. Consequences of mild deficiency in children. Extent and meaning of iron deficiency. In: USA Proceedings of Workshop of Food and Nutrition Board. National Academy of Sciences, Washington DC

Illingworth R S 1986 Anaemia and child health surveillance. Archives of Disease in Childhood 61: 1151–1152

Illingworth R S 1987 The development of the infant and young child, 9th edn. Churchill Livingstone, Edinburgh

Jacobson R S, Straker G 1982 Peer group interaction of physically abused children. Child abuse and neglect. Child: Care, Health and Development 8: 219–225

James W H 1980 Gestational age in twins. Archives of Disease in Childhood 55: 281–284

Jannoun L 1983 Are cognitive and educational development affected by age at which prophylactic therapy is given in acute lymphoblastic leukaemia? Archives of Disease in Childhood 58: 953–958

Jencks C, Smith M, Acland M et al 1973 Inequality: a reassessment of the effect of family and schooling in America. Allen Lane, London

Jonsson G 1967 Delinquent boys, their parents and grandparents. Acta Psychiatrica Scandinavica 43, Suppl 195

Keats J 1820 To Autumn

Kitchen W H 1978 The small baby. Short term and long term prognosis. Medical Journal of Australia 28: 82–84

Klaus M H, Jerauld R, Kreger N C, McAlpine W, Steffa M, Kennell J H 1972 Maternal attachment. Importance of the first post-partum days. New England Journal of Medicine 286: 460

Knobloch H, Pasamanick B 1974 Gesell and Amatruda's developmental diagnosis, 3rd edn. Harper & Row, Maryland, pp 244–246

Konishi Y, Kuriyama M, Mikawa H, Suzuki J 1987 Effect of body position on later postural and functional lateralities of preterm infants. Developmental Medicine and Child Neurology 29: 751–757

Lansdown R G et al 1974 Lancet i: 538

Lansdown R, Yule W 1986 The lead debate. The environment, toxicology and child health. Croom Helm, London

Lansdown R 1984 Child development. Made Simple Books, Heinemann, London

Largo R H, Pfister D, Molinari L, Kundu S, Lipp A, Duc G 1989 Significance of prenatal, perinatal and postnatal factors in the development of Aga preterm infants at five to seven years. Developmental Medicine and Child Neurology 31: 440–456

Lefebvre F, Bard H, Veilleux A, Martel C 1988 Outcome at school age of children with birthweights of 1000 grams or less. Developmental Medicine and Child Neurology 30: 170–180

Lester D 1967 The relationship between discipline experiences and the expression of aggression. American Anthropology 69: 734–737

Lewis C, Newsom E, Newsom J 1982 Father participation through childhood: the impact of the father. In: Beail N, McQuire J (eds) Fathers: psychological perspectives. Junction Books, London

Lindahl E, Michelsson K, Helenius M, Parre M 1988 Neonatal risk factors and later neurodevelopmental disturbances. Developmental Medicine and Child Neurology 30: 571–589

Lindsay J, Ounsted C, Richards P 1979 Long term outcome in children with temporal lobe seizures. 1. Social outcome and childhood factors. Developmental Medicine and Child Neurology 21: 285–298

Lloyd-Still J D 1976 Malnutrition and intellectual development. MTP Press, London

Lobo E deH 1978 Children of immigrants to Britain, their health and social problems. Hodder & Stoughton, London

Lorenz K 1970 Studies in animal and human behaviour. Harvard University Press, Cambridge, Massachusetts

Low J A, Galbraith R S, Muir D W, Broekhoven L H, Wilkinson J W, Karchmar E J 1985 The contribution of fetal-newborn complications to motor and cognitive deficits. Developmental Medicine and Child Neurology 27: 578–587

Lucas A, Morley R, Cole T J et al 1989 Early diet in preterm babies and developmental status in infancy. Archives of Disease in Childhood 64: 1570–1578

Ludman L, Lansdown R, Spitz L 1989 Factors associated with developmental progress of full term neonates who required intensive care. Archives of Disease in Childhood 64: 33–337

Luria A R 1932 The nature of human conflicts. Liverlight, New York

Maccoby E E, Jacklin C N 1980 Psychological sex differences. In: Rutter M (ed) Scientific foundations of developmental psychiatry. Heinemann Medical Books, London

Madge N, Tizard J 1980 Intelligence In: Rutter M L (ed) Scientific foundations of developmental psychiatry. Heinemann Medical Books, London

McNeil J L, Ptasnik J A 1974 International symposium on recent advances in the assessment of the health effects of environmental pollution. 24. Commission of the European Communities, Luxembourg

Michaels R H, Rogers K D 1971 A sex difference in immunologic responsiveness. Pediatrics 47: 121

Michelsson K, Ylinen A, Donner M 1981 Neurodevelopmental screening at five years of children who were at risk neonatally. Developmental Medicine and Child Neurology 23: 427–433

Minturn L, Lambert W W 1964 Mothers of six cultures. Wiley, New York

Mitchell R E 1971 Some social implications of high density housing. American Sociology Review 36: 18–29

Mittler P 1970 Biological and social aspects of language development in twins. Developmental Medicine and Child Neurology 12: 741–757

Montcrieff A A, Koumides O P, Clayton B E, Patrick A D, Renwick A G C, Roberts G E 1964. 1. Lead poisoning in children. Archives of Disease in Childhood 39: 1–13

Murphy G, Hulse J A, Jackson D et al 1986 Early treated hypothyroidism: development at 3 years. Archives of Disease in Childhood 61: 761–765

Murphy M, Botting B 1989 Twinning rates and social class in Great Britain. Archives of Disease in Childhood 64: 272–274

Murray-Lyon I M Adverse effects of alcohol in pregnancy. Gastroenterology in Practice June/July: 8–14

Neligan G A, Prudham D 1976 Family factors affecting child development. Archives of Disease in Childhood 51: 853–858

Newsom J, Newsom E 1963 Infant care in an urban community. Allen & Unwin, London

Newsom J, Newsom E 1968 Four years old in an urban community. Allen & Unwin, London

Nilsson N 1985 Children's play needs are international.

Ojofeitimi E O 1984 Assessment of the nutritional status of Nigerian rural children and mothers' perceptions of quality of life. Child: Care, Health and Development 10: 349–358

Osborn A F, Butler N R, Morris A C 1984 The social life of Britain's five-year-olds. A report of the Child Health and Education Study. Routledge and Kegan Paul, London

Paludetto R, Rinaldi P, Mansi G, Andolfi M, Del Giudice G 1984 Early behavioural development of preterm infants. Developmental Medicine and Child Neurology 26: 347–352

Parkinson C E, Wallis S M, Prince J, Harvey D 1982 Research note: rating the home environment of school-age children: a comparison with general cognitive index and school progress. Journal of Child Psychology and Psychiatry and Allied Disciplines 23.3: 329–333

Passow H H, Noah H J, Eckstein M A, Mallea J R 1976 The national case study. An empirical comparative study of twenty one educational systems. Almqvist & Wiksell, Stockholm

Phillips C J, Yuk-Ching H, Smith B, Sutton A 1986 Severe mental retardation in children from socially disadvantaged families. Child: Care, Health and Development 12: 69–91

Piper M C, Byrne P J, Darrah J, Watt M J 1989 Gross and fine motor development of preterm infants at eight and 12 months of age. Developmental Medicine and Child Neurology 31: 591–597

Plewis I 1981 Book review of nine year olds. Developmental Medicine and Child Neurology 23: 273–274

Plowden D 1967 Children and their primary schools, 2. Central Advisory Council for Education. HMSO, London

Pollak M, Tuchler H 1982 The Pollak Tapper. The Head Teachers' Review. 19–20

Pollak M, Mitchell S 1974 Early development of negro and white babies. Archives of Disease in Childhood 49: 40–45

Pollak M 1988 3 year olds around the world. Paper read at 1st International Conference of Social Paediatrics, Munich

Pollak M 1979 Housing and mothering. Archives of Disease in Childhood 54: 54–58

Portnoy S, Callias M, Wolke D, Gamsu H 1988 Five year follow-up of extremely low-birthweight infants. Developmental Medicine and Child Neurology 30: 590–598

Poskitt E M E, Hensey O J, Smith C S 1982 Alcohol, other drugs and the fetus. Developmental Medicine and Child Neurology 24: 596–602

Power M J, Benn R T, Morris J N 1972 Neighbourhood, school and juveniles before the courts. British Journal of Criminology 12: 111–132

Quinton D 1980 Cultural and community influences. In: Rutter M L (ed) Scientific foundations of developmental psychiatry, Heinemann Medical Books, London

Rantakallio P, von Wendt L 1985 Prognosis for low-birthweight infants up to the age of 14: a population study. Developmental Medicine and Child Neurology 27: 655–663

Report of the Central Advisory Council for Education (Chairman: Lady Plowden) 1967 Children and their primary schools. HMSO, London

Richards M 1982 Do broken marriages affect children? Health Visitor 55: 152–153

Richman N 1972 Individual differences at birth. Developmental Medicine and Child Neurology 14: 400–401

Richman N 1974 The effects of housing on pre-school children and their mothers. Developmental Medicine and Child Neurology 16: 53–58

Robinson A 1969 Sex differences in development. Developmental Medicine and Child Neurology 11: 245–246

Robinson R O 1977 Fetal alcohol syndrome. Developmental Medicine and Child Neurology 19: 538–539

Ross G, Lipper E G, Auld P A M 1987 Hand preference of four year old children. Its relationship to premature birth and neurodevelopmental outcome. Developmental Medicine and Child Neurology 29: 615–622

Rubin R A, Balow B 1980 Infant neurological abnormalities as indicators of cognitive impairment. Developmental Medicine and Child Neurology 22: 336–343

Rutter M 1980 The longterm effects of early experience. Developmental Medicine and Child Neurology 22: 800–815

Rutter M, Korn S, Birch H G 1963 Genetic and environmental factors in the development of 'primary reaction patterns'. British Journal of Social Clinical Psychology 2: 161–173

Rutter M, Yule B, Quinton D, Rowlands O, Yule W, Berger M 1975 Attainment and adjustment in two geographical areas. iii Some factors accounting for area differences. British Journal of Psychiatry 126: 520–533

Rutter M L, Madge N 1976 Cycles of deprivation. Heinemann, London

Rutter M L, Tizard J, Whitmore K 1970 Education, health and behaviour. Longman, London

Rutter M, Maugham B, Mortimore P, Ouston J 1979 Fifteen thousand hours. Open Books, London

Rutter M 1971 Parent–child separation: psychological effects on the children. Journal of Child Psychology and Psychiatry and Allied Disciplines 12: 233–260

Rutter M, Quinton D 1975 Psychiatric disorder: ecological factors and concepts of causation. In: McGurk H (ed) Ecological factors in human development. North Holland

Rutter M 1972 Maternal deprivation reassessed. Penguin, Harmondsworth

Sameroff A J, Chandler M J 1975 Reproductive risk and the continuum of caretaking causality. In: Horowitz F D, Hetherington M, Scarr-Salapatek S, Siegel G (eds) Review of child development research, 4. University of Chicago Press, Chicago

Sarsfield J K 1974 The neurological sequelae of non-accidental injury. Developmental Medicine and Child Neurology 16: 826–827

Saunders M 1977 A review of studies of the socio-familial backgrounds and educational facilities of the homes of moderately educationally subnormal children. Child: Care, Health and Development 3: 407–423

Scheiner A P 1980 Perinatal asphyxia: factors which predict developmental outcome. Developmental Medicine and Child Neurology 22: 102–104

Scott J P 1958 Critical periods in the development of social behaviour in puppies. Psychosomatic Medicine 20: 42

Scott S 1975 White and West Indian infants in London: development from birth to 44 weeks of age. Child: Care, Health and Development 1: 203–215

Shaffer D 1973 Psychiatric aspects of brain injury in childhood. Developmental Medicine and Child Neurology 15: 211

Shaffer D R 1985 Developmental psychology. Theory, research and applications. Brooks/Cole, Monterey, California

Shelter (SHAC) 1988 Prescription for poor health. Maternity Alliance London Food Commission, London

Shields J 1980 Genetics and mental development. In: Rutter M (Ed) The scientific foundations of developmental psychiatry. Heinemann, London

Showers J, McCleery J T 1984 Research on twins: implications for parenting. Child: Care, Health and Development 10: 391–404

Silva P A, McGee R O, Powell J 1982 Growth and development of twins compared with singletons at ages 5 and 7: a followup report from the Dunedin Multidisciplinary Child Development Study. Australian Paediatric Journal 18: 35–36

Skorodok L M 1969 The influence of substitutional hormone therapy on the mental development of hypothyroid children. Pediatrya 48: 81

Skouteli H N, Dubowitz L M S, Levene M L, Miller G 1985 Predictors for survival and normal neurodevelopmental outcome of infants weighing less than 1001 grams at birth. Developmental Medicine and Child Neurology 27: 588–595

Smart J G, Jeffrey C, Richards B 1980 A retrospective study of the relationship between birth history and handedness at 6 years. Early Human Development 4: 79–88

Smith J A, Wallace S J 1982 Febrile convulsions: intellectual progress in relation to anticonvulsant therapy and to recurrence of fits. Archives of Disease in Childhood 57.2: 104–108

Social Trends. A publication of the Government Statistical Service. HMSO, London

Sokol R J, Miller S L, Reed G 1980 Alcohol abuse during pregnancy: an epidemiologic study. Alcoholism: Clinical and Experimental Research 4: 135–145

Solomons G, Solomons H C 1975 Motor development in Yucatecan infants. Developmental Medicine and Child Neurology 17: 41–46

Spiers P S, Wacholder S 1982 Association between rates of premature delivery and intra-uterine growth retardation. Developmental Medicine and Child Neurology 24: 808–816

State of the World's Children. Published for UNICEF by Oxford University Press, Oxford

Stein Z, Susser M, Saenger G, Marolla F 1972 Intelligence test results of individuals exposed during gestation to the World War 2 famine in the Netherlands. Tijdschrift voor Soc. Geneeskunde 50: 766

Stein Z, Susser M 1960 Families of dull children. Parts 2, 3, 4. Journal of Mental Science 106: 1296–1319

Steiner E S, Sanders E M, Phillips E C K, Maddock C R 1980 Very low-birthweight children at school age: comparison of neonatal management methods. British Medical Journal 281: 1237–1239

Stewart A L, Costello A M deL, Hamilton P A et al 1989 Relationship between neurodevelopmental status of very preterm infants at one and four years. Developmental Medicine and Child Neurology 31: 756–765

Stores G 1971 Cognitive function in epilepsy. British Journal of Hospital Medicine 6: 207

Stores G 1978 School-children with epilepsy at risk for learning and behaviour problems. Developmental Medicine and Child Neurology 20: 502–508

Stott D H 1973 Follow up from birth of the effects of prenatal stress. Developmental Medicine and Child Neurology 15: 770–787

Sullivan W C 1899 A note on the influence of maternal inebriety on the offspring. Journal of Mental Science 45: 489–503

Super C M 1976 Environmental effects on motor development: the case of 'African infant precocity'. Developmental Medicine and Child Neurology 18: 561–567

Swan R W, Stavros H 1973 Child rearing practices associated with the development of cognitive skills of children in low socio-economic areas. Early Child Development and Care 2: 23–38

Sylva K, Lunt I 1982 Child development. A first course. Grant McIntyre, London

Sylva K 1989 Does early intervention "work"? Archives of Disease in Childhood 64: 1103–1104

Tada H, Wallace S J, Hughes I A 1986 Height in epilepsy. Archives of Disease in Childhood 61: 1224

Taylor B, Wadsworth J 1984 Breast feeding and child development at 5 years. Developmental Medicine and Child Neurology 26: 73–80

The Black Report 1980 Inequalities in health: report of a research working group. DHSS, London

Tizard B, Hodges J 1978 The effect of early institutional rearing on the development of eight year old children. Journal of Child Psychology and Psychiatry and Allied Disciplines 19: 99–118

Tizard B, Rees J 1975 The effects of early institutional rearing on the behaviour problems and affectional relationships of 4-year-old children. Journal of Child Psychology and Psychiatry and Allied Disciplines 16: 61–73

Tizard J, Plewis I 1977 Critical Notice. Preschool IQ: prenatal and early developmental correlates. Journal of Child Psychology and Psychiatry and Allied Disciplines 18: 381–388

Tizard J 1970 The role of social institutions in the causation, prevention and alleviation of mental retardation. In: Haywood H C (ed) Social–cultural aspects of mental retardation. Appleton-Century Crofts, London

Tucker D M, Sandstead H H, Penland J M, Dawson S L, Milne D B 1984 Iron status and brain function: serum ferritin levels associated with asymmetries of cortical electrophysiology and cognitive performance. American Journal of Clinical Nutrition 39: 105–113

Twaddle V, Britton P G, Craft A C, Noble T C, Kernahan J 1983 Intellectual function after treatment for leukaemia or solid tumours. Archives of Disease in Childhood 58: 949–952

Twaddle V, Britton P G, Kernahan J, Craft A W 1986 Intellect after malignancy. Archives of Disease in Childhood 61: 700–702

Tylor E 1889 Primitive culture. Holt, New York

Ueda R 1978 Standardization of the Denver Developmental screening test on Tokyo children. Developmental Medicine and Child Neurology 20: 647–656

Ultmann M H, Belman A L, Ruff H A, Novick B E, Cone-Wesson B, Cohen H J, Rubinstein A 1985 Developmental abnormalities in infants and children with acquired immune deficiency syndrome (AIDS) and AIDS related complex. Developmental Medicine and Child Neurology 27: 563–571

Viani F, Beghi E, Romeo A, van Lierde A 1987 Infantile febrile status epilepticus: risk factors and outcome. Developmental Medicine and Child Neurology 29: 495–501

Vince M A 1959 Effects of age and experience on the establishment of internal inhibition in finches. British Journal of Psychology 50: 136

Vohr B R, Garcia-Coll C, Oh W 1989 Language and neurodevelopmental outcome of low-birthweight infants at three years. Developmental Medicine and Child Neurology 31: 582–590

Wallerstein J S, Kelly J B 1975 The effects of parental divorce experiences of the preschool child. Journal of the American Academy of Child Psychiatry 14: 600–616

Waters B, Dimock J 1983 A review of research relevant to custody and access disputes. Australian and New Zealand Journal of Psychiatry 17: 181–189

Weisglas-Kuperus N, Uleman-Vleeschdrager M, Baerts W 1987 Ventricular haemorrhages and hypoxic-ischaemic lesions in preterm infants: neurodevelopmental outcome at 3 and a half years. Developmental Medicine and Child Neurology 29: 623–629

Westin-Lindgren G 1982 Achievement and mental ability of physically late and early maturing schoolchildren related to their social background. Journal of Child Psychology and Psychiatry and Allied Disciplines 23.4: 407–420

White Franklin A 1975 Concerning child abuse. Churchill Livingstone, Edinburgh

WHO/Marga Institute 1984 Intersectorial action for health. Sri Lanka study. Colombo, Sri Lanka

Wilson R S 1981 Mental development: concordance for same-sex and opposite sex dizygotic twins. Developmental Psychology 5: 626–629

Winter S T 1972 The male disadvantage in diseases acquired in childhood. Developmental Medicine and Child Neurology 14: 517–520

Winter S T, Mainzer W 1962 Factors in the hospitalization of Haifa children. Israel Medical Journal 20: 143

Wise P H, Koelchuck M, Wilson M L, Mills M 1985 Racial and socioeconomic disparities in childhood mortality in Boston. New England Journal of Medicine 313: 360–366

Yatkin V S, McLaren D S 1970 The behavioural development of infants recovering from severe malnutrition. Journal of Mental Deficiency Research 14: 25–32

Yule W, Lansdown R, Millar I B, Urbanowicz M 1981 The relationship between blood lead concentrations, intelligence and attainment in a school population: a pilot study. Developmental Medicine and Child Neurology 23: 567–576

Zeskind P S, Ramey C T 1981 Preventing intellectual and interactional sequelae of fetal malnutrition: a longitudinal, transactional and synergistic approach to development. Child Development 52: 213–218

Zubrick S R, Macartney H, Stanley F J 1988 Hidden handicap in school age children who received neonatal intensive care. Developmental Medicine and Child Neurology 30: 145–152

Zuckerman B S, Hingson R 1986 Alcohol consumption during pregnancy: a critical review. Developmental Medicine and Child Neurology 28: 649–661

Zur J, Yule W 1990 Chronic solvent abuse. 1. Cognitive sequelae. 2. Relationship with depression. Child: Care, Health and Development 16: 1–34

4. History-taking and medical examination

The proper study [of medicine] is of the patient who happens to have a disease and not the disease which the patient happens to have.

[William Osler]

HISTORY-TAKING

An accurate history has been and remains one of the cornerstones of clinical medicine and is as true of developmental paediatrics as of other branches of medicine with the difference that the major part of the history is given by parents rather than the patient.

Some estimate of the accuracy of the witness is required and the unreliability of parents' memory for past developmental milestones has been recorded (Hart et al 1978). The longer the time between the passing of the milestone and the enquiry the less accurate the answer is likely to be. Immunization status and birth events are both subjects about which parents have been shown to have poor memories (Nicol et al 1987). This inaccuracy is more likely to apply to *normal* child development: parents — and grandparents — are more precise about developmental delays or abnormalities and remember the time at which they became worried about an unattained milestone, etc.

The condition presented to the developmental paediatrician (DP) is likely to be both chronic and complicated; the patient unlikely to be acutely and gravely ill. A thorough enquiry of past history is required and whether progression or regression has occurred. Time taken in good history gathering is well spent as this is probably the first meeting of child, parents and paediatrician. Time is also needed for parents to air worries; the child and paediatrician to develop friendly relations and the doctor to observe the child/parent relationship. It is important that this first interview between the three parties is a successful one. Firstly the doctor will be in a better position to gain the child's cooperation in the ensuing examination; secondly the doctor has to rely upon the quality of the relationship forged between the parents and himself to gain a cooperative response to any treatment and counselling prescribed possibly over several ensuing years.

The importance of noting what parents say needs no emphasis but there are exceptions. Child and sexual abuse and Munchausen Syndrome are three examples of subjects on which parents do not readily offer information. Sometimes the subject is not thought important or, if they suspect their child is mentally retarded, they may be sparing with the truth or antedate developmental milestones. So direct questions about, for example, hospital admissions, accidents, myopia, strabismus and language delay, etc. may be asked. A parent is very unlikely to state he/she blames him/herself or the marital partner or that the marriage is under great strain although both marital partners may have such thoughts. The DP needs to exercise judgement by specifically raising such questions so parents discuss a subject which they felt unable to spontaneously. Such questions are not to be construed as judgemental; on the contrary, to suggest to parents that such feelings are normal and they are not alone in having such thoughts.

An overall plan of history taking will include: the child, parents, family life and the child's environment. Although the DP allows parent(s) ample opportunity to convey anxieties, they need guiding through history taking in a way that allows the physician to gather the information in an orderly fashion.

The child is *never* forgotten. Asking a child his own ideas always proves interesting and sometimes is more accurate and reliable than information from parents! For example, parents are sometimes slow at noticing signs of depression in their children (Angold et al 1987). And, even if the history is not accurate, the problem can be seen through the child's eyes. Children are usually very honest about their relationships with the family, siblings in particular. Many are very open in either accepting or disagreeing with their parents' judgements of them. There is no reason why a child should not be present whilst the parent gives their history nor why the child cannot be asked his view of any behavioural problems mentioned. He probably has his own opinion.

In considering the presenting symptom(s) answers can be sought to the following questions:

— why has it been presented at this particular time ?
— has the condition deteriorated?
— are the parents at their wits' end because of behaviour problems?
— have they had help or battled on alone?

The child

Ante- and perinatal history

A search will be made for risk factors, e.g. threatened miscarriage, bleeding during pregnancy, prematurity, low birthweight (<1500 g), small-for-dates, neonatal respiratory failure and hypoxia from other causes. Most mothers know the reason for early induction of labour, caesarean section or forceps delivery but it is useful to look at the obstetric and neonatal notes if available. Of what importance and relevance are any abnormalities discovered?

Low birthweight and prematurity. For the majority of babies of low birthweight and gestational age the outcome is good but it will be remembered that the smallest amd most immature babies are those most likely to suffer major impairments. Approximately 10% of low birthweight babies weighing less than 1500 g at birth but whose weight is appropriate for gestational age will have developmental disabilites at 3 years (Ross et al 1986). 29% of babies less than 33 weeks' gestation, if assessed at 4 years, are likely to have neurodevelopmental problems of which 15% are major. The latter problems will include neurological movement problems, sensorineural hearing losses and epilepsy (Costello et al 1988, Lindahl et al 1988). Approximately one-third of low birthweight babies will have 'unsatisfactory progress' at school (Rickards et al 1988). Children who are small-for-dates at birth and whose head growth slowed before 26 weeks' gestation achieve less well at school than normal birthweight children (Parkinson et al 1981). More than 50% of spastic diplegia, the more common type of cerebral palsy which accounts for one-third of cases (Pharoah et al 1987), will have been born prematurely (Cooke 1990) and an adverse pre- or perinatal history is likely when VLBW babies develop spastic diplegia (Wild et al 1988). The low birthweight baby who develops cerebral palsy is likely to have a spastic diplegia which has less involvement of the upper limbs and is associated with less mental retardation than diplegics of normal birthweight. (Drillien et al 1962). Atkinson (1983) concluded that the likelihood is that LBW babies are damaged in utero whilst the NBW group are brain-damaged as a result of traumatic births. A premature birth means that an allowance in the early months has to be made in the developmental assessment.

Respiratory problems. Hypoxia with hypertonia may be associated with brain damage (Brown et al 1974). Of babies requiring ventilatory support for more than 48 hours, about 10% at 2 years will have major disabilites attributable to their neonatal status (Mali et al 1989). 7% of babies who had mechanical ventilation for neonatal respiratory failure will have a major handicap. The very small babies are the worst affected and those with perinatal asphyxia (Gunn et al 1983).

Combination of neonatal risk factors. Late language may be associated with multiple neonatal risk factors (Zubrick et al 1988, Lindahl et al 1988, Gunn et al 1983). There is *no* evidence that fullterm jaundiced babies who receive phototherapy later show developmental delays (Telzrow et al 1980). The likelihood of babies who suffer haemolytic disease in the newborn period and receive exchange transfusion suffering any later developmental damage is remote (Walker et al 1974).

Early thriving and growth

Being small. Weight, height and head circumference are affected by being born small-for-dates. Normally these dimensions show a sex difference, with boys increasing to a greater degree in all three than girls. But born small-for-dates babies of both sexes show a proportional greater increase in head circumference than babies of normal gestation (Ounsted et al 1982). A false impression of head charts may be formed unless this is known. Being small is associated with later psychological and social behavioural aberrations (Skuse 1987). Learning problems are more common in small children (Gold 1978). Failure to thrive is associated with retardation of growth and behaviour problems and the average IQ of such children may be depressed (Skuse 1985). Failure to thrive may be due to a young and inexperienced mother and may occur in the babies of Asian mothers who are insecure, socially isolated and whose husbands do not accept there is a problem (Fenton et al 1989). Rarely, congenital myasthenia presents as a feeding difficulty with weak sucking and swallowing but ptosis, hypotonia and external ophthalmoplegia will create a suspicion of neuromuscular disorder.

Developmental milestones

General developmental delay. Delayed milestones in all parameters with motor milestones the least affected.

Expressive language delays and learning problems. When part of a generalized neuro-developmental delay, are associated with a history of delay in motor milestones and late toilet training.

Language delay. A history will be obtained of all three aspects of language development. Whether this is a bi- or tri-lingual family and whether there has been a succession of different language speaking au-pairs? Questions will be asked to establish whether there is language delay or disorder (see Ch. 9).

Congenital hearing loss. In addition to a history of language development, the possibility of lip reading and gesturing sought. A history of play is also helpful.

Motor milestones. In cases of motor delay and suspected neurological abnormality motor milestones will be delayed. Creepers and shufflers are likely to be late walkers and there may well be a positive family history (Robson 1970).

Illnesses and medical conditions

Many medical conditions are relevant to a child's developmental progress and the following are the more common:

Head injury. Head injuries in childhood may result in significant intellectual impairment, especially visuospatial skills, the severity of which is related to length of unconsciousness and presence of cerebral oedema (Rutter et al 1980). 23% of children aged 4–10 years with severe brain injury and unconsciousness were unable to attend normal schools and a further 25% were functioning below their previous levels (Heiskanen & Kaste 1974). The age at which the injury is sustained does not appear to matter (Chadwick et al 1981). Generalized damage commonly causes general intellectual impairment whilst local trauma causes the appropriate neurological deficits (Heiskanen & Kaste 1974).

Non-traumatic coma. This can cause developmental delay and is directly related to the severity of the coma on admission and condition during the ensuing 24 hours (Seshia et al 1983).

Accidents. These have a developmental history (See Ch. 2). Ingestions and lacerations reflect the mobility of the child. Older children can clamber and climb and will ingest the contents of cupboards or burn or scald themselves with electric fires or matches (Fig. 4.1). Immobile babies are more likely to ingest articles close at hand and be scalded by pulling things over themselves.

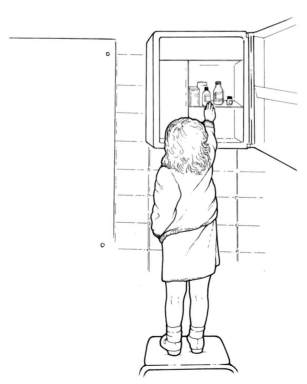

Fig. 4.1   Mobile and climbing up to cupboard.

Infections

Encephalitis and meningitis. Associated with impaired brain function and the earlier they are sustained the greater is the likelihood of damage (Sells et al 1975).

Viral infections. Those of the CNS are mostly benign in character (Seshia et al 1983) but children, all of whom had suffered the infection under 1 year of age, were found to be 6 points lower on performance (WISC) tests compared with matched controls when tested at least 5 years after the infection (Chamberlain et al 1983).

Meningitis. If extending through the CSF into the labyrinth, can cause a permanent sensorineural hearing loss and is the most common cause of postnatal hearing loss amongst school-age deaf children. Deafness is particularly associated with the suppurative type of meningitis. Approximately 80% occurs in children under 5 years, half of whom are under 2 years. Previously, the impairment of hearing was compounded when ototoxic agents were used as therapy. Meningitis in the neonatal period has the most serious prognosis and approximately 10–20% of *all* types of neonatal meningitis who survive have neurological handicaps (Hull et al 1981) although figures as high as 25–38% have been quoted (Catlin 1978). No nerve deafness was found in children who had suffered gram-positive neonatal meningitis but 73% had delayed speech and language development and 44% were functioning at less than average intellectual functioning (Fitzhardinge et al 1974). *H. Influenzae* meningitis, the most common type of meningitis, is well known to cause severe, often bilateral, hearing loss. In 1971/2 30% of children with the infection had complications of hearing (Gamstropp & Klockhoff 1974) but the incidence has fallen, with improved treatment schemata. Aseptic types of meningitis, e.g. those due to tubercle bacilli, carry a high risk of sequelae which include cerebral palsy, epilepsy and optic atrophy.

Approximately 4–8% of cases of encephalitis following *mumps* can cause unilateral sensorineural deafness. *Measles encephalitis* may cause deafness and serious neurological handicaps with impaired mental function. Survivors of herpes encephalitis often suffer mental impairment.

Seizure disorders — infantile spasms, fits, epilepsy

It may be better to think of epilepsy as a symptom rather than a discrete entity and in young children seizures are best thought of developmentally, according to the age at which they occur. The younger the baby or child the worse the prognosis, although an uncommon but benign form of neonatal seizure has been described (Verity 1988).

Infantile spasms. These are serious and have a grave prognosis despite early treatment with steroids. In a follow-up of 98 children at least 5 years after their initial attacks, two-thirds had had further fits and half had a neurological abnormality (Jeavons et al 1970). A Japanese study was even more depressing. Only 10% of children had made a complete recovery. The poor outcome for the rest resulted in poor physical development and mental retardation. A preceding history of perinatal risk factors or poor development exacerbated the poor prognosis (Matsumoto et al 1981). Associated neonatal hypopituitarism carries a poor prognosis as most continue to have seizures and associated mental retardation (Costello et al 1988). In another study, 28% on follow-up were suffering from psychiatric disorders of which half were diagnosed as infantile autism (Riikonen & Amnell 1981).

Febrile convulsions. Have a much more benign outcome, only one-third suffer a further attack and most follow-ups report no serious sequelae (Costeff et al 1982, Schottz-Christensen et al 1973) and many none at all (Verity et al 1985, Nelson et al 1978). If a child remits, his/her sibling has a 38% risk of a seizure (Lindsay et al 1980).

Epilepsy. Classification of epilepsies is problematic. Children not only have different types of seizures, as shown on the EEG, but the same child, especially if suffering the myoclonic type, may have different types of fits at different times. Children with epilepsy have a higher rate of psychiatric disorders than either healthy children or children with other handicaps (Rutter et al 1970). This rate is increased by the site of the lesion, an adverse reaction to treatment and psychiatric instability in the family (Stores 1978). Epileptics (febrile and single childhood fits excluded) with a mean age of 33 years were divided into those who were 'uncomplicated' (idiopathic) and 'complicated'. It was found that both types had a higher mortality than controls. The complicated types had lower educational and social achievements than the uncomplicated who were more like the average population (Britten et al 1986).

Studying epileptic children at ordinary schools, Holdsworth & Whitmore (1974) discovered 16% were falling seriously behind in their scholastic studies and 21% had deviant behaviour, frequency of fits being an important factor in the latter. Inattentiveness applied to both groups. Focal epilepsies, carefully selected and treated by neurosurgery had a good prognosis with improved school achievements and personalsocial behaviour (Lindsay et al 1980, 1984). Lennox-Gastaut and myoclonic types of epilepsy are associated with mental retardation (Tassinari 1985).

Malnutrition

The effects of malnutrition have been described in Chapter 3. Unfortunately there is no agreement about sequelae amongst experts. Children who had been grossly undernourished and marasmic in the first two years of life, 20 years later were significantly lower in height, weight and intelligence (Stoch et al 1982) but these were not the findings of Grantham-McGregor et al (1982). Other factors, such as child abuse, nonorganic failure to thrive and vulnerable child syndrome may be involved in those children who do not make marked improvement (Dixon et al 1982). The sequelae of malnutrition are unclear and faced with a history of malnutrition in children from underdeveloped countries the clinician will have to exercise clinical judgement as to how important the history is to any clinical findings.

Spina bifida

A crucial factor in a patient with spina bifida is whether a shunt was needed to control the hydrocephalus because the necessity for a shunt is likely to affect developmental outcome. Spain (1974) found only one-third of children with shunts were developing normally scoring less than average on performance scores. 3-year-olds also had lower verbal scores despite their hyper-verbality. Memory function has also been found to be poor (Cull & Wyke 1984). Children who have shunts for post-haemorrhagic ventricular dilatation appear to have a grave prognosis. 25% of two-year survivors had quadriplegia and severe mental retardation. Only 25% were normal (Hislop et al 1988). Tew & Laurence (1983) reported a group of schoolchildren with hydrocephalus some of whom were shunt-controlled and some were not. The mean IQ of both was at the lower end of average. The stability of their IQs throughout their school lives was noted.

Child abuse

Delicate questioning may be required to produce correct answers; asking whether the family have a social worker may be a good entree. Incidence is higher in handicapped children. Although not well researched at present, the likelihood of later developmental problems is high and consequences serious. Up to 30–45% of abused children suffer from mental retardation. Elmer & Gregg (1967) estimated that 25% have cerebral damage and 50% may be mentally retarded. The same authors reported 42% developmentally retarded. Damage is related to the type of injury suffered, mental retardation being more common following a fractured skull or subdural haemorrhage. Speech delays, reading retardation, learning and behavioural problems are common sequelae and occur in children who have not suffered head injuries (Oates et al 1984).

Lead poisoning

High levels of lead pollution in the environment have been correlated with lower scholastic achievements and (possibly) cognitive function (Fergusson et al 1988). Serious permanent neurological damage including optic atrophy has been described (Betts et al 1973) and in a recent study in northern Italy lead levels in teeth were directly related to WISC-R IQ scores (Bergomi et al 1989). However the evidence of developmental damage following raised blood lead levels remains conflicting (Baltrop 1976).

Duchenne muscular dystrophy

Developmental impairments in patients with Duchenne dystrophy have included: lower IQ (Karagan 1979); language deficits (Karagan et al 1980); word finding ability (Leibowitz & Dubowitz 1981); motor skills (Sollee et al 1985) and reading skills (Dorman et al 1988).

Acquired immune deficiency syndrome (AIDS) and AIDS-related complex

Children suffering these conditions are known to have delayed developmental milestones especially in motor development. Cognitive function is also subnormal. Some children with AIDS have lost achievements as the illness has progressed (Ultmann et al 1985).

Chromosomal abnormalities Fragile X and 47XXY karyotypes

It is now claimed that the high incidence of Fragile X makes it the second most common genetic cause of mental retardation (Down syndrome being the first) (Winter 1989). Boys suffering from 47XXY karyotype abnormality may have problems of personalsocial development including timidity, lack of confidence, impaired sexual development and social competence (Bancroft et al 1982)

Some medical conditions of early childhood which might have been expected to affect developmental progress but which do *not* are: congenital hypothyroidism which receives early treatment (Murphy et al 1986); epilepsy which does not appear to affect linear growth (Tada et al 1986); chronic childhood asthma is not associated with delay in growth but with a delay in puberty (Balfour-Lynn 1986).

Parents and family life

Demographic data of the family gives a picture of the life which the patient is living, family size and the ages of other children. Consanguinity may be important in families from the Middle and Far East. Social class, past educational achievement and the presence of any familial or genetically acquired disease are relevant. The DP will make some estimate of the intelligence of the parents since many developmental conditions are associated with low IQ in parents. Hess et al (1977) equated a lower maternal IQ with children suffering failure to thrive for nonorganic reasons. These factors are important not only in estimating the effect of family and events on the child but also in the planning and ultimate success of long-term treatment and care. Both parents will be interviewed if possible. They may have differing views of the presenting problem and this is an opportunity to make an appraisal of their relationship; their acceptance or rejection of the child and his symptoms. It may be relevant to notice the fathers who insist on coming and those who never come. If granny comes as well — beware!

Maternal history

Age. There is a high prevalence of *trisomy 21 (and other trisomies)* amongst children born to mothers over 35 years of age and a relationship between rising maternal age and *mental retardation* in their babies (Tizard & Grad 1961); dyslexia (Street & Jayasekara 1978); autism (Gillberg 1980); fine-motor problems, visuo-perceptual dysfunction and attentional deficit have all been found to increase in the children of mothers of a mean age of 39.4 years compared with children whose mothers had a mean age of 27.9 years (Gillberg et al 1982).

Parity. High parity is related to perinatal mortality and thus with increased developmental disabilities (Kirman 1977).

Illnesses during pregnancy. A number of infections, such as rubella and cytomegalic toxoplasmosis, have effects on development. Maternal urinary infections and low birthweight have been associated (Naeye 1979).

Breast feeding. Fergusson et al (1987) have effectively quashed any reported association between breast feeding and conduct disorders.

Depression. Having three or more children under 14 years of age; being within 3 months following childbirth; caring for a young child, especially one who is handicapped, are all factors which increase the likelihood of a mother suffering from depression (Richman 1976). The effects which maternal depression is likely to have on her child's development are: an increase in behaviour problems, especially preschool children (Wolff 1961, 1986); delayed expressive language (Cox et al 1987) and an increased likelihood of physical abuse (Richman 1975).

Alcohol. The effect of alcohol consumption during pregnancy has been discussed in Chapter 3. In the presence of dysmorphic facies and mental retardation questions will be asked about alcohol consumption during the pregnancy. Whether the answer is reliable will be for the clinician to decide! It would possibly be more reliable to ask the child. Children as young as 6 years old have an extremely accurate idea about alcohol and their parents' excessive drinking habits (Ritson 1975; Pollak 1979).

Smoking and drugs taken during pregnancy. Smoking has been associated with low birthweight (Meyer 1978). Some drugs are thought to affect the fetus. The list is long (Smith 1976).

and Moslems between whom there was no real difference (Checuti et al 1985). There is some disagreement about the applicability of Western height and weight charts to children of Asian and Far Eastern ethnic minorities (Pollak 1989) but most studies refer to children in their own countries and not their progress in the UK. It is the child's progressive deviation from his own original centile which is important and it is satisfactory to chart this on standard charts. A study of schoolchildren in Leeds, of whom approximately 10% were ethnic minorities, concluded that the Tanner growth charts were applicable to all the children (Buckler 1985). However the *weight* of Asian and Bangladeshi infants approximates more to the 25th percentile than the 50th on Tanner-Whitehouse scales (Davies & Wheeler 1989). There may be a difference in the growth of hands in different countries (Flatt & Burmeister 1979). Several studies have confirmed there is no difference in the mean heights and weights of children with sickle cell trait and West Indian children with normal haemoglobins (Ashcroft et al 1969, 1978). There is no apparent relationship between menarche and body size in developed countries (Stark et al 1989).

Height

During the 1970s an increase occurred in the mean height of children (boys more than girls) in the UK and standard measurements have come under review (Voss 1987). Owing to an increase in the multicultural mix in the UK in the previous years it was necessary to see whether the current charts could be applied equally to different ethnic groups. Children of Afro-Caribbean origin were taller than Caucasian children (Chinn et al 1989). The majority of children of short stature are small because one (or both) of their parents is small. If the height of the child is plotted and compared with that of the father and mother it can be seen whether his height falls within the expected range or not (Tanner et al 1970). Many medical conditions are associated with short stature and some of the more common are:

1. **Chromosomal abnormalities**
   Down's syndrome
   XO Turner syndrome (usually normal at birth) (Fig. 4.4).
   This patient is 23 years old.

2. **Intrauterine maldevelopment**
   Fetal alcohol syndrome
   Russell-Silver syndromes
   Cornelia-de-Lange syndrome
   Prader-Willi syndrome (may also be obese).

3. **Skeletal abnormalities**
   Achrondroplasia
   Hurler syndrome

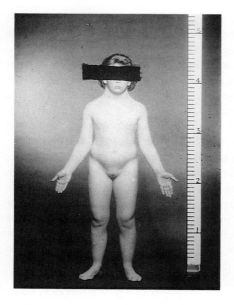

Fig. 4.4   Turner syndrome, aged 23 years (Courtesy of the Gordon Photographic Museum, Guy's Hospital).

Osteogenesis imperfecta
Rickets
Still's disease.

4. **Endocrine abnormalities** associated with pituitary or hypothalamic dysfunction
    Adrenal hyperplasia (Young et al 1989)
    Laurence-Moon-Biedl syndrome
    Hypothyroidism
    Cushing syndrome.

5. **Miscellaneous**
    Glycogen storage disease
    Thalassaemia
    Coeliac disease
    Any condition causing protein and calorie deficiency
    Emotional child abuse
    Cerebral palsy
    Some infections, e.g. meningitis, toxoplasmosis.

Myelomeningocele is associated with a growth deficit resulting in short stature. The higher the level of the meningocele, the greater the growth defect. This is more marked in the legs and Rosenblum et al (1983) found that many patients had longer armspan than expected. Prediabetic metabolic abnormality enhances skeletal maturity in both sexes and this skeletal maturity continues to operate in girls after treatment despite a reduction in growth rate but this does not apply to boys (Edelstein et al 1981). Whether growth charts are applicable to some children with an intrinsic growth disorder has been questioned (Hulse 1988) and the growth patterns of achondroplasia (Horton et al 1978), Turner's syndrome (Pelz et al 1982, Lyon et al 1985) and Klinefelter's syndrome (Schibler et al 1974, Caldwell & Smith 1972) have been researched. Readers are advised to study these. There are special charts for young Down syndrome children (Cronk et al 1988).

In some patients with chronic diseases and malnutrition, growth can *slow down* and, when the cause has been lack of food, if corrected, *catch-up growth* can occur. Catch-up growth also occurs after treatment with thyroid and growth hormones and has been described after removal of an adrenal tumour. Babies with coeliac disease or pyloric stenosis may catch-up after treatment. Children with cerebral palsy who had gastrostomies for poor growth have been described as improving following the operation (Shapiro et al 1986). Poor growth associated with child abuse can be followed by catch-up growth when the children are taken into long-term fostercare (King & Taitz 1985). During catch-up times charts will not be applicable. Almost normal catch-up growth occurs in prenatal growth retardation of late pregnancy which arises in an otherwise normal fetus. This is seen in twins (Prader 1978). When weight, height and head circumference of small-for-dates babies are measured the head circumference, especially that of boys, catches up more than the two other measurements (Ounsted et al 1982). Do very low birthweight babies catch up? Long-term survivors who weighed between 1000 and 1500 g at birth were measured when they were 8 years old. Three-quarters of the *small* for gestational age babies had a height (and weight) above the l0th percentile. Almost none who were *appropriate* for gestational age were below the 10th (Kitchen 1980). VLBW babies, with appropriate weight for gestational age, were followed up at 2 years: 71% had caught up but, of 29% who remained below the 10th percentile in weight, there was a much higher incidence of major and minor developmental disabilities (Astbury et al 1986). There is a relationship between lower educational achievement and significant growth retardation (below the 5th percentile) (Holmes et al 1984); height and weight and short stature irrespective of cause (Dowdney et al 1987). Goldstein (1987) demonstrated a significant positive relationship between skeletal age and cognitive development (controlled for chronological age) in 12–17-year-olds.

Head circumference

Head circumference is measured by a nonstretchable tape measure over the maximum circumference around the occipital protuberance and the supraorbital ridges (Fig. 4.5) and the position on the percentile charts is then plotted. A sensible deduction from the measurement of the head circumference is made when taken in conjuction with measurements of height and weight as the three have a relationship to each other. A large

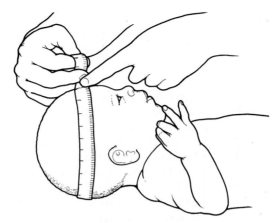

Fig. 4.5   Measuring head circumference.

baby can be expected to have a large head. Some gifted individuals such as Napoleon, Byron and Bismarck have had large heads but many have not. Day & Schutt (1979) studied 15 normal children with large heads (>0.5 cm above the 98th percentile) and in 13 cases made a diagnosis of benign familial megalencephaly. Although Grantham-McGregor & Desai (1973) found the heads of male babies born in Kingston, Jamaica grew more quickly during the first 3 months of life than expected from international standards, this rapid growth, which also applied to height and weight, slowed after 3 months and there was no difference by one year. Nevertheless Nellhaus (1968) does not consider there are geographical or racial differences in head circumference. No differences in these measurements are reported in several racial groups (Nelson & Deutschberger 1970). As Illingworth (1987) points out, if the brain does not grow neither does the head and, on average, mentally retarded children have smaller heads than children of average intelligence. This is more likely to apply to mental retardation present from birth or the first year of life. Mental retardation of later onset is likely to be associated with a head of normal proportions.

A distinction is made between a large head (macrocephaly) and a large brain (megalencephaly), the latter term being reserved for large head which is not hydrocephalic.

Macrocephaly is associated with hydrocephalus, subdural effusion, space-occupying lesion or thickened skull.

Megalencephaly is applied to cerebral degenerative conditions, achondroplasia and neurofibromatosis but most cases are of unknown aetiology or familial.

557 children referred in childhood because of a large head (cases of spina bifida being excluded) were reviewed 20 years later; 20% were dead and 70% of those alive had raised intracranial pressure, 20% had large

recognizable genetic, metabolic, chromosomal or neurological basis to the retardation whilst an IQ above 60 is unlikely to have identifiable signs. Hence further investigations are more likely to be warranted for the latter. (See proviso in Ch. 13.)

2. Might the disorder be genetic in origin? If so, and the condition is severe, this would be an indication for further investigations. It would be reasonable and humane to offer parents genetic counselling.

3. It is natural that parents faced with a mentally retarded child wish to know the reason for it. Their secret hope is that the retardation is unconnected with them and they suffer from a mixture of denial, guilt and depression. Their marital relations may be under strain. The DP has a duty to make an assessment of the severity of this position and on this basis may consider the advisability of further investigations because of the (remote) possibility of making a correct diagnosis.

4. Some of the investigations outlined below require interpretation by an expert in the field and need an expert's opinion upon the indication for it. Therefore the DP needs to know his limitations and when to refer or obtain a second opinion.

A combination of all these four factors can help the DP make a decision as to the advisability of further investigations which may include:

- *Urine studies* for reducing substances, ketones, aminoacids and polymucosaccharides.
- *Serological tests* for antenatal infections, when indicated.
- *Chromatography* for urea, uric acid and amino acid.
- *Skin biopsy.* Sometimes enzymes can be quantified in leucocytes or fibroblasts.
- *Thyroid hormone estimation.* X-rays of the *skull* can show calcification (e.g. toxoplasmosis, cytomegalovirus infection, Sturge-Weber syndrome), a space-occupying lesion or increased pressure. Unfortunately X-rays are usually unhelpful. Occasionally X-rays of *long bones* may show up mucopolysaccharidosis. The skull can be transilluminated to show fluid collection and, occasionally, cerebral atrophy. *Bone age* can be used to estimate physiological age, growth potential and adult stature; diagnosis of growth hormone and thyroid deficiency; metabolic disorders of growth and monitoring treatment (Buckler 1983, Tanner et al 1975).
- *Chromosomal investigations.* These may include *buccal smears* which are microscopically examined for X and Y chromatin material; *skin biopsies* and *amniotic fluid* which allow karyotype analysis of leucocytes or fibroblasts. An influential paper by Thake et al (1987) used chromosome studies of children in ESN(M) and ESN(S) schools in Coventry. 16% of moderately mentally handicapped children were found to have the fragile X syndrome of whom 37% were boys and 63% were girls. These studies revealed two other important findings.

Firstly, twice as many children who were positive for the fragile X were moderately retarded as were severely retarded. Secondly the occurrence of mental retardation in a sibling was 1:2 for boys and 1:4 for girls. The authors suggest that in both sexes large ears and IQs in the 50–70 range are useful signs of suspicion of this condition and a head circumference and testicular volume above the 50th percentile in males.

- *Electroencephalography (EEG)*. This investigation is most commonly used in children with a history of convulsions. There is a very wide range of normal in children which makes the interpretation of border-line abnormalities the province of the expert. Maturation changes in the EEG bear some relationship to the maturation of cerebral tissue. Abnormal seizure discharges can be demonstrated in some cases and a complex, mixed pattern, occurring in clusters, is characteristic of infantile spasms. (Of course, the differential diagnosis of infantile spasms itself is complex.) EEG and polygraphic recordings in the newborn have a prognostic significance for developmental and neurological outcome (Karch et al 1984).

- *Computerized axial tomography (CAT)*. CAT has revolutionized the study of the brain. The test needs the child to remain still for several minutes so sedation or anaesthesia is required but the manoeuvre is noninvasive. A computer analyses different densities of different tissues. It is specially valuable in hydrocephalus and intraventricular haemorrhage. Cysts and tumours are defined and so it may prove helpful in some difficult cases of epilepsy. Brain atrophy following 'the shaken infant syndrome' has been demonstrated (Frank et al 1985) and changes in white matter show up before they become calcified. The use of this device in revealing congenital malformations is only beginning to be realized. In expert hands, the technique can differentiate between megalencephaly, extraventricular hydrocephalus and communicating hydrocephalus (Gooskens et al 1988). CAT can also be used for other areas of the body. Bleck (1984) describes its use in the diagnosis of children's hips. Unfortunately, currently in the UK it is not widely available and very costly. But, with increased availability, it will eliminate the need for invasive procedures such as myelography, cerebral angiogram, etc.

- *Isotope brain scanning* can give a picture of CSF flow and is useful in monitoring subdural effusion, vascular anomalies, neoplasms and abscesses.

- *Nuclear magnetic resonance (NMR)*. NMR can define brain damage and is especially useful in the newborn as ionizing radiation is not required. Although developed by a British doctor, Britain is singularly lacking in this most useful equipment which reduces dependence on radiation whilst visualizing the human body in the transverse plane.

- *Neuromuscular function tests*. Neuromuscular disorders may be investigated by *creatine phosphokinase (CPK)* estimation — the level being quick procedures and a time commitment has to be made to obtain an accurate assessment.

Who should perform this assessment?

Knobloch & Pasamanick (1963) stated: 'the physician has the responsibility for diagnosing developmental status, particularly in infancy, and he cannot delegate this responsibility to someone else'. There *is* a case for the initial assessment being made by one clinician because of the following advantages:

1. There is no need to 'cut up' the child into a developmental and a neurological half. The neurological examination can start by, for example, the child catching a ball, walking or hopping and can appear as an extension of the 'games'.

2. By mixing in tests of hearing, vision and medical examination with the developmental assessment, the child is not upset. Undressing the child completely is usually unnecessary if clothes are pulled up or down. When full undressing *is* necessary, bit-by-bit and redressing as soon as possible is more successful; if the child does it himself whilst the examiner kneels on the floor beside the plastic mat the situation is least threatening.

3. Judgement and assessment can be made at every turn. Examples are:

— Does the child only respond if you shout?
— Does he lip read?
— Although silent, does he complete non-verbal tasks well?
— Is apparent clumsiness accompanied by inspecting material at a small focal range? (The author has a vivid memory of Dr. Ronnie MacKeith saying it is no good assessing the motor and neurological status in great detail if one has failed to note that he tripped over the carpet because he did not see it.)
— Does he understand what is expected of him?
— Does his mother repeatedly try to help him because she knows that he cannot do the task and she does not want you to know?
— When shyness is overcome, is speech good for age?
— As each examination is completed, the examiner gains confirmation or otherwise of his initial suspicion of diagnosis.
— The examiner can decide which, from a variety of tests, will be most suitable for the next parameter to be examined.
— If the clinician decides the child *can* but *will not* undertake the task, the examiner can use every wile until co-operation is obtained. This saves the child and his parents the need to attend on different occasions. The child only needs to be 'acclimatized' once which helps both in gaining and keeping his attention. Rona et al (1987) found that attention and concentrations difficulties were the most common

problems encountered in the developmental examinations and were the most common reason for noncompliance.

— the DP gains experience in assessing the whole child. By mixing, matching and comparing all the various parameters and combining these with medical, auditory, visual and neurological examinations, the DP can make a diagnosis based on a knowlege of all factors which may affect development.

The method described above uses the developmentalist as the 'overall' screener. He can then consult with or refer to his appropriate specialist colleague(s) either for their further detailed examination or directly for treatment. An advantage to other specialist members of the Child Development Centre team is that they are not used as screeners for every patient and their expert knowledge is used only where it can be best employed. A disadvantage is that it demands considerable expertise.

TEST OF DEVELOPMENTAL ASSESSMENT

Which tests should be used?

There is a plethora of tests, almost all of which derive either from Gesell's original work or the neurodevelopmental tests described by Brazelton et al (1969), Prechtl & Beintema (1964), Touwen (1976) and Rutter et al (1970). Developmental tests available can be divided into three main types:

Screening tests
Scale type tests
Clinical tests.

Screening tests

Denver developmental screening test (DDST) (Frankenburg & Dodds 1967)

The most well-known screening test, the DDST is in wide use and the scales have been used successfully by health visitors and other health workers as well as doctors. The best use of DDST is as a screening test of normality when 94% reliability can be expected (Greer et al 1989). However, it has been criticized as a predictive measure, Greer et al concluding that 80% of children who later had a poor outcome were not identified. It is not suitable, therefore, for developmental assessments.

Scale type tests

Bayley Scales of Infant Development (Bayley 1969)

This is an American test which covers from birth to $2\frac{1}{2}$ years. It takes 45 minutes to complete. There are three scales:

Mental scales yielding a mental development index (MDI)
Motor scales yielding a psychomotor development index (PDI).
Infant behaviour scales which are observational and judgemental and have no score.

The two indices can be computed into a single index and the scales give an indication of a child's current functioning. The scales have limited value as predictors of later abilities and Bayley (1969) conceded it is not possible to compute index scores for profoundly handicapped children, a situation confirmed in a study by Chech & Gallagher (1985) in which normal and abnormal babies were compared on these scales and the Chicago Infant Neuromotor Assessment (CINMA). The scales had validity in normal babies but the latter were more sensitive in abnormal infants. Significant differences have been reported in the results of babies from different cultures (Solomons 1975, Solomons 1978).

Griffiths Scales of Mental Development (Griffiths 1954, 1970)

This is a British test for children from 2–8 years and takes about one hour to administer. There are five subtests:

Locomotor
Personalsocial
Hearing and speech
Hand-eye coordination
Performance
Practical reasoning is added for 3–8-year-olds.

Each subtest gives a developmental quotient (DQ) which is averaged into a general quotient (GQ). The quotients are based on mental age scores and have been successfully used in cross-cultural studies, e.g. UK and Brazil (Victoria et al 1990). Only measurements of mental ages can be used in handicapped children. Inter-rater reliability on eye-hand coordination, performance and practical reasoning is high but locomotor, personalsocial and hearing-speech scales are less reliable (Smith et al 1980). A minor discrepancy of inter-rater scoring for mental age particularly in younger age groups can lead to a very wide discrepancy in the developmental quotient (Smith et al 1980). Many test items, even in as important a parameter as language, rely upon the mother's (or caregiver's) replies to questions. Hanson et al (1984) gave this as the main reason for differences in scores which were reached by 10 observers watching the same 6 videotapes. The same authors (1987) describe changes in mean general quotient between 1960 (100.4) and 1980 (111.7). Social classes showed wide variations — classes 1 and 2 a mean GQ of 121 and classes 4 and 5 a GQ of 106. The authors conclude the scales have limited value for children with normal GQs over 4 years of age. Scores on the Bayley scales are consistently lower than similar tasks on the Griffiths Scales (Ramsay & Fitzhardinge 1977, Beail 1985) so comparisons cannot be made.

Both the Bayley and Griffiths scales are suitable for second-level screening of preschool children. They are of very limited value as serial records of handicapped children.

Brazelton neonatal behavioural assessment scale (NBAS) (Brazelton, 1973)

These scales examine the intactness of a neonate on a four-point scale of 20 reflex items; the scales were reviewed and a second edition issued 10 years later which greatly extended their scope (Brazelton 1984). There are 28 standard items, nine items for 'fragile' babies and 18 elicited responses which consist of known neurological reactions. Follow-up studies have not yet been published. These scales have pushed the assessment of the behaviour of infants into the newborn period and are extremely valuable for this reason; for example, Als et al (1976) found the NBAS was effective in differentiating fullterm babies who were underweight from those of full weight.

Clinically based tests

1. Gesell schedules

Gesell's work has been described in Chapters 1 and 2. His book *The First Five Years of Life* (1954) describes the developmental parameters in detail whilst *'Developmental Diagnosis'* (Gesell & Amatruda 1941) describes child development at different age ranges and normal and abnormal child development. Tests of development are described in detail at 'key' ages in the former and paediatric applications and clinical methods in the latter. Gesell's basic concepts remain the foundation on which most other tests and schemes have been built. Gesell did not see his schedules as screening devices and stressed the clinical nature of his work. In the preface to the first edition, Gesell writes, 'this book is the fruit of a *clinical loom'*. Normal, atypical and abnormal child development are given equal weight. His developmental norms are based on extensive work with normal children and often observed two children of the same age together. The developmental parameters were first described in 1925 and divided into:

- Motor
- Personalsocial
- Adaptive
- Language.

The basic structure of the developmental norms and parameters has stood the test of time. Although much work has been done and published since 1925, these have been essentially refinements and subdivisions rather than any major reorganization.

Table 5.2 Scoring system for external criteria (From Dubowitz L M S, Dubowitz V, Goldberg C. Clinical assessment of gestational age in the newborn infant. Journal of Pediatrics 1970 77:1–10, adapted from Farr and associates Developmental Medicine and Child Neurology 1966 8:507)

External sign	Score 0	1	2	3	4
Oedema	Obvious oedema of hands and feet; pitting over tibia	No obvious oedema of hands and feet; pitting over tibia	No oedema		
Skin texture	Very thin, gelatinous	Thin and smooth	Smooth; medium thickness. Rash or superficial peeling	Slight thickening. Superficial cracking and peeling especially of hands and feet	Thick and parchment-like; superficial or deep cracking
Skin colour	Dark red	Uniformly pink	Pale pink; variable over body	Pale; only pink over ears, lips, palms, or soles	
Skin opacity (trunk)	Numerous veins and venules clearly seen, especially over abdomen	Veins and tributaries seen	A few large vessels clearly seen over abdomen	A few large vessels seen indistinctly over abdomen	No blood vessels seen
Lanugo (over back)	No lanugo	Abundant; long and thick over whole back	Hair thinning especially over lower back	Small amount of lanugo and bald areas	At least half of back devoid of lanugo
Plantar creases	No skin creases	Faint red marks over anterior half of sole	Definite red marks over anterior half; indentations over anterior third	Indentations over anterior third	Definite deep indentations over anterior third
Nipple formation	Nipple barely visible. No areola	Nipple well defined; areola smooth and flat, diameter 0.75 cm	Areola stippled, edge not raised, diameter 0.75 cm	Areola stippled, edge raised diameter 0.75 cm	
Breast size	No breast tissue palpable	Breast tissue on one or both sides, 0.5 cm diameter	Breast tissue both sides; one or both 0.5-1.0 cm	Breast tissue both sides; one or both 1 cm	
Ear form	Pinna flat and shapeless, little or no incurving of edge	Incurving of part of edge of pinna	Partial incurving whole of upper pinna	Well-defined incurving whole of upper pinna	
Ear firmness	Pinna soft, easily folded, no recoil	Pinna soft, easily folded, slow recoil	Cartilage to edge of pinna, but soft in places, ready recoil	Pinna firm, cartilage to edge; instant recoil	
Genitals: Male	Neither testis in scrotum	At least one testis high in scrotum	At least one testis right down		
Female (with hips half abducted)	Labia majora widely separated, labia minora protruding	Labia majora almost cover labia minora	Labia majora completely cover labia minora		

Adaptive development

The case for starting any developmental assessment with bricks has already been made and other nonverbal tests such as formboards, spatial puzzles and drawing follow. Almost all children, regardless of ability, enjoy these tests. Children with a language disorder or autism who apparently have no communicating skills, will cast darting glances towards nonverbal material. Their problem is eye-to-eye contact rather than disinterest in inert material and they often surprise by their performance. Whilst measuring adaptive development the examiner can note the fine manipulative skills with which the child has carried out the tasks, pencil grasp for example.

Vision

Nonverbal tasks may be conveniently followed by matching letters and vision testing. Use of the Stycar letter cards or the Sonksen-Silver tests (see Ch. 12) are those most suitable for this age group. Some children, especially in the 2-year age group, are bored by matching a letter to the one on their card. This can be overcome by one of two methods. Either the examination starts with the 6/6 size letters and, only if an incorrect result for each eye separately and together is obtained, are the larger size letters used, or encouragement to flagging interest is given by flipping over the cards at a very quick rate. Visual acuity will not be the only visual test. The eyes will be observed for unilateral differences and ptosis; eye movements are tested; the presence of strabismus, overt or latent, sought, as is nystagmus. Clinical examination of the peripheral fields is rarely productive in the absence of gross neurological abnormality but all handicapped children should have their visual fields carefully mapped out.

Language development

Symbolic language. One of the reasons for starting with nonverbal tests is that many young children are reluctant to talk early on in the assessment, especially when they have a language problem or are shy. However, their achievement in nonverbal tests will encourage them and it is rare that they are not talking by this stage. However, it is advantageous to start assessing language development by a test of *symbolic language*. The Making-Tea-Test (Pollak 1972) is an example and almost all children will take the proffered toys. The meaningfulness and maturity of their actions is the reason behind the test and ability to symbolize the toys is shown by the child's unconscious use of them. Children may offer their mother, themselves or the examiner the imaginary cup of tea, all of which are less mature reactions than giving the teacup to the miniature dolls. Their clumsy attempts to place the dolls on the tiny chairs may exasperate them and they throw the whole test on the floor! More than symbolic language is examined since any tremor or clumsiness is very apparent and it is a test of fine manipulative skill to seat the tiny doll upon the miniature chair. Throughout the assessment the examiner is weighing up whether, taking all other aspects into account, the child has behaved to an appropriate level.

Comprehension and expression. The Reynell developmental language scales (RDLS) (Reynell 1969) are a suitable first choice since children enjoy these scales and the developmental phases through which the children are taken are accurate. An age level is obtained for both comprehension and expression and the percentile charts are useful as criteria for intervention and comparison at follow-up. The tests of expression of the RDLS are less good and the Renfrew word finding test cards (Renfrew 1972) may be substituted despite the fact that a few of the pictures are old-fashioned. The Reed hearing test card (Royal National Institute for the Deaf) is an alternative.

By this stage the DP will know whether there is a serious problem of language, in which case Bishop's Test for the reception of grammar (TROG) (Bishop 1977) will be the next choice (see Ch. 9). If a child is unable to undertake the language tests successfully, or there is obvious serious delay, the test of symbolic language is repeated. If the results of this, as well as those of adaptive development, are low this is highly suggestive that the child has poor mental abilities. A lower score in language development than adaptive suggests a language problem and/or deafness.

Hearing

If a language problem has been found, exclusion of a hearing loss is necessary and tests of hearing described in Chapter 11 can be carried out next. Objective tests are best for making the differential diagnosis with audiometry and tympanometry the methods of choice.

Motor development

The child has been sitting at his table until this stage and changing to physical activity makes a welcome change. It may well start with throwing a large ball (made of sponge for obvious reasons!) and throwing and catching maturity measured. When examining children with short attention spans and poor concentration who are threatening noncooperation, a sudden switch to ballplay may please the child and regain his cooperation.

Motor development will 'slide' into the neurological examination and the two can be combined in this age group. *Locomotor* development is examined by running, hopping and jumping. *Balance* is tested by line or

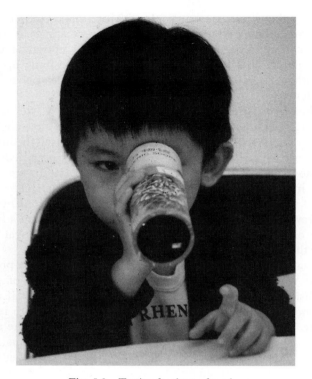

Fig. 5.2   Testing for the preferred eye.

beam walking on one or both legs and control in different positions. *Limb, hand and eye preference* (Fig. 5.2) and any asymmetry is noted. Gross motor development will also be tested. *Fine motor skills* have already been noted in the manipulation of test material, particularly pencil hold, and can also be noted if the child takes off his coat or shoes and socks for testing reflexes.

Neurological examination

Gestures and other movement patterns are tested and, when tendon-reflex testing follows, most of the essentials of a neurological examination of a child of this age will have been completed. Movements of the tongue and the finger-nose test may be included. The motor and neurological intactness of children with language deficits as well as the mentally retarded and any child with a congenital abnormality require examination. From these results the paediatrician is now in a position to decide whether there is a neurological basis to the developmental diagnosis.

Table 5.3 Developmental profiles for children aged 1–5 years according to handicap

	Motor		Adaptive
	Gross	Fine	
Mild mental retardation without other handicap	N	MD	D
Severe mental retardation without physical handicap	MD	D	D or P
Mild language delay	N	N or MD	N
Severe language delay	N	N or MD	N
Language disorder	N	N	N or MD
Congenital deafness	N	N	N or MD
Acquired deafness, normal IQ	N	N	N
Congential blindness	MD	MD	MD
Partial sight, normal IQ	N	MD	N
Mild cerebral palsy, normal IQ	D or P	D or P	N
Severe cerebral palsy, normal IQ	P	P	D
Normal IQ, severe environmental deprivation	N	N	N

N = normal; MD = mild delay; D = delay; P = pathological.

REFERENCES

Als H, Trionick E, Adamson L, Brazelton T B 1976 The behavior of the full-term but underweight newborn infant. Developmental Medicine and Child Neurology 18: 590–602
Amiel-Tilson C, Stewart A 1989 Follow up studies during the first five years of life: a pervasive assessment of neurological function. Archives of Disease in Childhood 64: 496–502
Andre-Thomas C Y, Saint-Anne Dargassies S 1960 The neurological examination of the infant. Medical Advisory Council/National Spastics Society, London
Bax M, Whitmore K 1987 The medical examination of children on entry to school. The results and use of neurodevelopmental assessment. Developmental Medicine and Child Neurology 29: 40–55
Bayley N 1969 Bayley Scales of Infant Development. The Psychological Corporation, New York
Beail N 1985 A comparative study of profoundly multiply handicapped children's scores on the Bayley and the Griffiths developmental scales. Child: Care, Health and Development 11: 31–36
Bellman M H, Rawson N S B, Wadsworth J, Ros E M, Cameron S, Miller D L 1985 A developmental test based on the Stycar sequences used in the National Childhood Encephalopathy Study. Child: Care, Health and Development 11: 309–323
Bene E, Anthony J 1978 Family relations test: an objective for exploring emotional attitudes in children. NFER–Nelson, Windsor
Birch H, Lefford A 1963 Intersensory development in children. Monographs of the Society for Research in Child Development 28: 89
Bishop D M 1977 Test for the reception of grammar (TROG). NFER–Nelson, Windsor
Brazelton C B, Robey J S, Collier G A 1969 Infant development in Zinacanteco Indians of Southern Mexico. Pediatrics 44: 274–290
Brazelton T B 1973 Neonatal behavioural assessment scale, 1st edn. Clinics in Developmental Medicine 50. Spastics International Medical Publications/Heinemann Medical Books, London

Table 5.3 (contd)

Language				Personalsocial	
Symbolic	Comprehensive	Expressive	Articulate	Personal	Social
D	D	MD	MD	D	D
D	D	D	D	D	D
N	N	D	MD	N	N
N	D	D	D	N	D or P
P	P	P	D	D	P
MD	D	P	P	N or D	D
N	D	P	P	N	Shy
MD	N	MD	N	D	D
N	N	MD	N	N	N
N	N	MD	MD or P	N	N
D	MD	D	D	D	D
N	MD	D	MD	N	MD

Brazelton T B 1984 Neonatal behavioural assessment scale, 2nd edn. Clinics in Developmental Medicine 88. Spastics International Medical Publications/Heinemann Medical Books, London

Caron A J, Caron R F 1982 Cognitive development in early infancy. In: Field T M, Huston A, Quay H C, Troll C, Finley G (eds) Review of Human Development. Wiley, New York

Carr J, Stephen E 1964 Paediatricians and developmental tests. Developmental Medicine and Child Neurology 6: 614–620

Chamberlain R, Davey A 1976 Cross-sectional study of developmental test items in children aged 94–97 weeks: report on the British Births Child Study. Developmental Medicine and Child Neurology 18: 54–70

Chech D, Gallagher R J 1985 Infant motor assessment — Bayley scales of infant development compared with Chicago Infant Neuromotor assessment.

Cooper J, Moodley M, Reynell J 1978 Helping language development: A developmental programme for children with early language handicaps. Edward Arnold, London

Dargassies S 1972 Neurodevelopmental symptoms during the first year of life. Developmental Medicine and Child Neurology 14: 235–246

Drillien C M, Pickering R M, Drummond M B 1988 Predictive value of screening for different areas of development. Developmental Medicine and Child Neurology 30: 294–305

Dubowitz L M S, Dubowitz V, Goldberg C 1970 Clinical assessment of gestational age in the newborn infant. Journal of Pediatrics 77: 1–10

Dubowitz L M S, Leibowitz D, Goldberg C 1977 A clinical screening test for assessment of intellectual development in four- and five-year-old children. Developmental Medicine and Child Neurology 19: 776–782

Dunn L M, Dunn L M 1981 Peabody Picture Vocabulary Test — revised. American Guidances Services, Circle Pines, Minnesota

Egan D F, Brown R 1984 Developmental assessment: 18 months to four and a half years. The Bus Puzzle Test. Child: Care, Health and Development 10: 163–179

Egan D, Brown R 1986a Developmental assessment: 18 months to 4 and a half years. Performance tests. Child: Care, Health and Development 12: 339–349

Egan D, Brown R 1986b Developmental assessment: 18 months to 4 and a half years. The miniature toys test. Child: Care, Health and Development 12: 167–181

Evans R, Ferguson N 1974 Screening school entrants. Journal of the Association of Educational Psychologists 3: 6

go through the one-foot and then two-foot takeoff and landing, and arms from behind to the mature forward swing.

Hopping

By $3\frac{1}{2}$ years most children can hop on their preferred leg for 3–6 steps. The number of steps and speed increase with age but children are 6 or 7 years old before voluntarily and rhythmically hopping on alternate feet.

Skipping

This is a complex variation of forward hopping, usually seen at 5 or 6 years of age (Fig. 6.2).

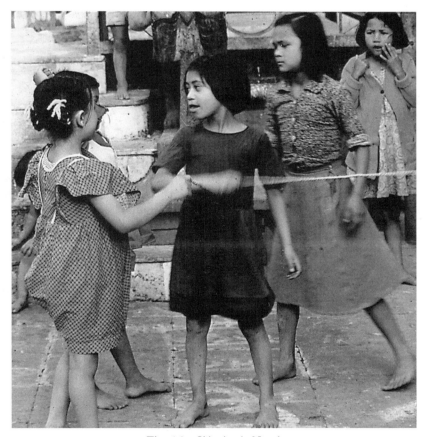

Fig. 6.2   Skipping in Nepal.

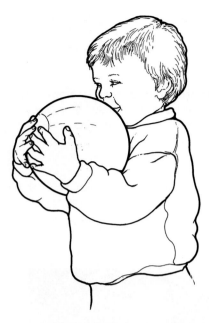

Fig. 6.3   'Cradling' the ball.

Throwing and catching

Throwing begins at *2 years* with underarm throwing with a relatively stiff body and no weight shift. *By $3\frac{1}{2}$ years* children rotate their bodies with the throw and *at 5 years* there is a mature throw with body swing and shift of weight and perhaps a short step forwards. A large ball is easier to throw than a small one.

Catching goes through developmental stages. Initially, it is merely an attempt to 'cradle' the ball against the body (Fig. 6.3) but by *4 years* the catch is anticipated by extending arms with little flexion of the elbows and feet together. By *5 or 6 years* he moves forwards towards the ball with one foot in front of the other, arms bent to catch the ball with both hands. Catching a bounced ball is a more difficult skill, as is catching with one hand only (preferred hand), the latter being a *9-year* achievement.

Balance

By 3 years of age children can stand momentarily on one leg; on tiptoe (both feet together) and walk in a straight line. By *4 years* they can walk in a circle and balance with one foot in front of another for 8–10 seconds. By *6 years* they can balance on one leg and one foot on tiptoe.

Thus babies develop from immobile, horizontal human beings into upright creatures capable of walking in any direction, running, jumping, standing on one leg and on tiptoe, with control, speed and strength developing (Denckla 1974).

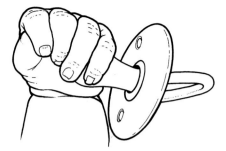

Fig. 6.4   Held with three ulnar fingers.

DEVELOPMENT OF FINE MANIPULATION

Hands and fingers are capable of extremely varied and complex movements and skills involving strength, speed, eye-motor coordination and perception.

Hand grasp and release

At birth hands are clenched and the grasp reflex may be strong enough to lift up the whole baby. *By 2 months* clenching lessens, fingers can be opened, occasionally spontaneously. At *3–4 months* if an object is placed in the hand it will be held with the 3 ulnar fingers in a (Fig. 6.4) largely involuntary action, the other hand simultaneously grasping. Release or reaching out are not yet possible but *by 5 months* the grasp reflex can be inhibited and objects released. There is a radial palmar grasp which includes thumb and index finger, i.e. whole hand grasp. Poor differentiation of hand and arm means that the elbow moves with the hand. The baby reaches out and picks up a toy, often examining his own hand and the toy alternately. *At 6 months*, with only one object in sight, reaching out and picking up is good with no simultaneous movement of the other hand. The wrist moves independently of the elbow. Fingertips are used for manipulation. Transfer of a cube from one hand to another occurs although release is primitive compared with grasp. Thus a brick may be put into a cup but not taken out as he cannot release it. At *6–7 months* old, a child has a good pincer grasp with forefinger and thumb and by *8 months* takes a proffered cube into either hand bringing the hands together in midline. *By 9 months* release is well developed and he throws everything out of the pram! His newly acquired object permanence is displayed by looking to see where it has fallen. A brick, placed under a cup whilst he looks, is found by lifting the cup. He pokes with outstretched index finger and points to distant objects. By *10–12 months* a cube is taken out of a cup and released by putting it back in. *By 14 months* one cube is put upon another and released. The height of the cube tower increases with increasing manipulative control but is not an increase in developmental skill.

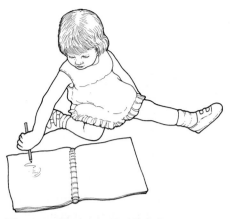

Fig. 6.5   Whole hand holding the pencil (outward).

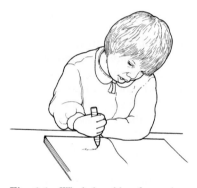

Fig. 6.6   Whole hand but forward grasp (midshaft).

Pencil holding

The first hold involves the whole hand which is often turned out, the whole arm moving the pencil, the hand only holding the pencil with correspondingly crude results (Fig. 6.5). The second hold is a 'whole hand' grasp (Fig. 6.6). The child begins to notice that extension of the index helps control and the wrist acts separately from the arm which is coming lower (Fig. 6.7). Finally the pencil has an adult hold with the arm on the table (Fig. 6.8). The development of the dynamic tripod has been described by Rosenbloom & Horton (1971) for ages 18 months and 7 years. Some further changes described in 7–14-year-olds suggests that maturation continues in the early school years (Ziviani 1983).

A little girl on the banks of the Nile had never seen a pencil before but after demonstration instinctively used this supinate grasp at midshaft (Fig. 6.9). She

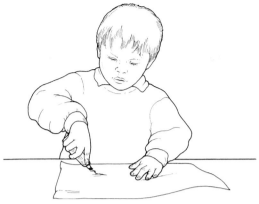

Fig. 6.7 Index finger beginning to give control.

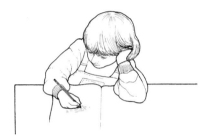

Fig. 6.8 Dynamic tripod grip.

was 29 months old. Rosenbloom suggests the age for this grasp is 28–30 months. Maturation of the neuromuscular system could be argued as the reason for the emergence of this motor skill since environmental factors had not caused any delay in this little girl's case.

Spoon and fork

Holding the grip on spoon and fork goes through the same stages as pencil holding and their use should be taught in the correct developmental phases.

Other hand movements

Many movements of the hands are possible and are acquired in developmental stages. Finger-to-thumb apposition and rapid alternating supination and pronation of forearms and hands both show developmental progression (Grant et al 1973). Finger-to-thumb apposition is mature by 7

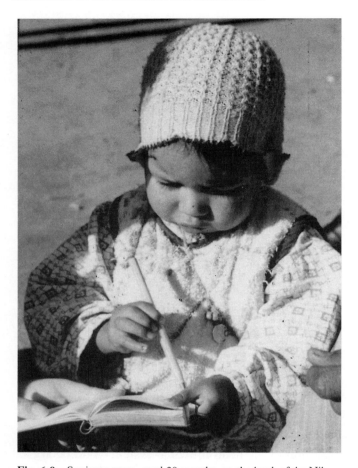

Fig. 6.9 Supinate grasp, aged 29 months, on the bank of the Nile.

years and pronation by *8 years*. *3-year-olds* can twist lids off bottles but not on again. This is the level for Caucasian children but in my experience *3-year-old* Vietnamese and Chinese children were well able to do both manoeuvres skilfully. Cutting with scissors is a complex skill and not acquired until *6 years* (Holle 1976) but this 4-year-old in a Vietnamese refugee camp in Hong Kong is already expert (Fig. 6.10). That not all artists are good developmentalists is shown by Figure 6.11, depicting the Three Wise Men paying homage to the newborn Child who can miraculously extend the two first fingers — a movement impossible to normal mortals until the age of 14 months! Elliott et al (1984) make a classification of manual manipulation based on function. Development of fine manipulation is demonstrated by the hand movements in catching a ball. Firstly, the hands 'cradle' the ball; then are cupped under the ball and the final mature grasp is with fingers outstretched.

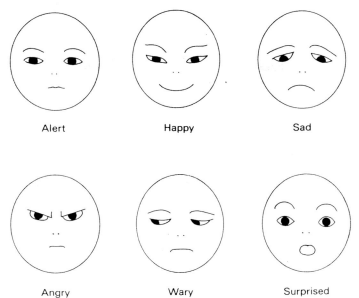

Fig. 6.12   Facial expressions (From Sheridan M D 1977 Observations on the development of spontaneous tele-kinesic communication in babies and young children. Child: Care, Health and Development 3:189–199. Courtesy of Blackwell Scientific Publications, Oxford).

and short are understood but 'longer' or 'shortest' not until *5 years*. Piaget (1970) has written extensively about the development of a child's concept of movement and speed which he divides into sensori-motor, intuitive and finally operational. Coordination of factors for skilled performance of motor skills thus develops during the first 18 months of life. Many of these factors are absent, abnormal or interfered with in lesions of upper motor neurones (e.g. cerebral palsy) and presumably partly account for the abnormal postures, tone and coordination seen in these conditions.

Mental retardation

Stages of motor development are usually delayed in *mental retardation* although less so than other parameters. Late head control delays other milestones including visual development, reaching out and fine manipulation. Mental retardation delays walking, although in the absence of motor disability most retarded children walk eventually. The age of walking is related to intelligence. Patients with an IQ above 50 walked before 4 years whilst those with an IQ below 50 (excluding children with cerebral palsy) walked by 8 years (Donoghue et al 1970). Children with Down syndrome are notably hypotonic in early childhood, and characterized by poor motor skills and stereognosis when older (Seyfort et al 1979), findings thought to be due to the reported diminution in size of the cerebellum in Down syndrome (Crome & Stern 1967).

Perinatal risk factors

Perinatal risk factors, including low Apgar score, limpness, apnoeic attacks and convulsions, have been associated with lower than average scores at age 6 on the Stott test and executive language scores (Jensen et al 1988). Delayed crawling and walking (compared with controls) were found in babies with no major neurological sequelae who had been in neonatal ICUs (Bottos et al 1989). The risk of neurological abnormalities in babies whose perinatal period was abnormal and who are late walkers is approximately 56% (Johnson et al 1990).

Extremely low birthweight

Opinion is divided as to the effect of *extremely low birthweight* on motor development. A recent study (Marlow et al 1989) of babies weighing less than 1251 g at birth reviewed their motor development at 6 years of age and all were considered to be neurologically normal but on the Henderson et al (1984) revision of the Stott the indexed children scored significantly less well on seven of the eight tests.

Prematurity

Does being born *preterm* per se affect early motor development or is the infant merely younger developmentally than the fullterm baby? There are adherents to both views — McGrew et al (1985) and Amiel-Tilson (1980) to the former; Gesell (1933) and Prechtl (1979) to the latter. In a study (without controls) Piper et al (1989) found differences in primitive reflexes but not in development of tone and voluntary movements which, if verified, give support to the developmental theory of maturity.

Muscle tone

Any condition markedly altering muscle tone is likely to affect motor development. The extensor hypertonia from which many children with cerebral palsy suffer prevents head control which, in turn, delays rolling over, sitting and walking. Unless and until primitive reflexes disappear many motor milestones cannot be reached. Tone in the upper limbs is often more normal than in the legs, and the child moves along the floor in 'commando' style (i.e. by flexion and extension of upper arms and dragging lower limbs along). Robson (1984) has predicted milestones for locomotion in children with hemiparesis and diplegia (Tables 6.1a and b, Tables 6.2a and b). Since asymmetry is one of the most important factors which influence locomotor strategies hemiplegics with one-sided loss of tactile sense are late in crawling and walking.

Table 6.1(a)   Hemiparesis/crawl type, predicting walking (to nearest half-month) (from Robson P 1984 Prewalking locomotor movements and their use in predicting standing and walking. Child: Care, Health and Development 10: 317–330, by courtesy of Blackwell Scientific Publications)

Stand	Walk ($\pm$2.5)	Correlation 0.72
6	7.0	
8	9.5	
10	12.0	
12	14.5	
14	17.0	
16	20.0	
18	22.5	
20	25.0	

Table 6.1(b)   Hemiparesis/shuffle type, milestones (in months) (from Robson P 1984 Prewalking locomotor movements and their use in predicting standing and walking. Child: Care, Health and Development 10: 317–330, by courtesy of Blackwell Scientific Publications)

Shuffle	Walk ($\pm$3.7)	Correlation 0.68
9	16.5	
11	18.5	
13	20.0	
15	22.0	
17	24.0	
19	25.5	
21	27.5	

Table 6.2   Diplegia/crawl type, predicting walking (to nearest half-month) (from Robson P 1984 Prewalking locomotor movements and their use in predicting standing and walking. Child: Care, Health and Development 10: 317–330, by courtesy of Blackwell Scientific Publications)

Stand	Walk ($\pm$2.5)	Correlation 0.86
9	14.0	
11	15.5	
13	17.0	
15	19.0	
17	21.0	
19	23.0	
21	25.5	
23	28.0	
25	31.0	
27	34.5	

Table 6.2b   Diplegia/shuffle type, predicting walking (to nearest month) (from Robson P 1984 Prewalking locomotor movements and their use in predicting standing and walking. Child: Care, Health and Development 10: 317–330, by courtesy of Blackwell Scientific Publications)

Shuffle	Walk (± 15.0)	Correlation 0.58
9	28.0	
13.0	34.0	
17.0	40.0	
21.0	46.0	
25.0	52.0	
29.0	58.0	
33.0	64.0	
37.0	70.0	
41.0	76.0	
45.0	83.0	

Vision

Vision is important in righting and orientation and when defective affects motor function. An inability to *fixate* or the presence of *strabismus and/or nystagmus* may delay motor development and affect balance. A high proportion of children with motor disturbances of cerebral origin have an associated strabismus. The reverse is not true and it has been postulated that, if the motor dysfunction of the squinting child were measured and found to be deficient, this might indicate that the strabismus was associated with neurological disorder. Postural sway and gait were tested and found to be deficient in squinting children compared with controls and it is suggested that both squint and motor deficit have a common central origin (Odenrick et al 1984). Clumsy children are reported to have a high degree of associated strabismus (Rasmussen et al 1983). In a study of 74 clumsy children who had reading and spelling problems 21% had a visual problem (6/12 or worse in one eye, 6/9 in both eyes or a treated or untreated squint).

Labyrinthine sense

A disturbance of labyrinthine sense will result in difficulties of balance and changing direction.

Joint sense

Any condition which restricts joint movements will affect gross motor development, movement and fine manipulation if hand and finger joints are involved.

cases where the righting reflex is absent passive standing attempted too early may frighten the child. The child with hemiplegia develops a typical arm and leg posture (Fig. 6.17).

The motor handicap of hemiplegics evolves round two problems — the equinus position of the ankle and difficulties with intricate hand function. Brown et al (1987) demonstrated decreased power and speed on the hemiplegic side with increased muscle tone and phasic spasticity on stretch. Children with spastic cerebral palsy show less ankle dorsiflexion and medial arch reactions than normal beginning walkers (Gunsolus et al 1975).

Abnormal hand and finger development

The clenched palms of the newborn may fail to relax after 12 weeks of age, making opening of the palms impossible. In hemiplegics there is a difference between the two hands making this an early diagnostic sign. Severe hyperextension, as seen in severe spastic cerebral palsy, causes the hand, when attempting to grasp an object, to take a position of extension

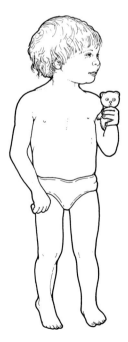

Fig. 6.17   Typical posture of hemiplegic.

at the wrist with the fingers splayed out in extreme extensor tone (Fig. 6.18). It is impossible for such a hand to grasp the object. Mentally retarded children may be late in developing hand regard, the normal stage of development being 3–5 months of age. Finger poking and pointing do not develop when fingers are incapable of individual movements.

Abnormal movement

Some children of low intelligence show *stereotypes* or rhythmic and repetitive movements, usually head-rolling, head-banging, rocking or waving the fingers against light. Stereotypes are sometimes seen briefly in normal children as a passing phase. Mentally retarded children may indulge in these movements for hours on end. Stereotypic movements are more common in young children, and gradually disappear although sometimes continue into adolescence (Mitchell et al 1977). Their aetiology is unknown although theories abound. The children derive some pleasure and possibly stimulation from their performance.

Late walkers

What is meant by late walking? Approximately 3% of 18-month-old children are not walking independently. Late walkers are a mixed group. In many a diagnosis is already known. For example, in Oxfordshire, 38% of children not walking at 18 months had cerebral palsy; 26% congenital syndromes and 14% mental retardation (without other signs). All were known abnormalities. The incidence of previously undetected neurological abnormality was 5.9% (Chaplais 1984). It is therefore well worth examining late walkers. In a follow-up study of babies who either weighed less than 2000 g at birth or who had been in the special care

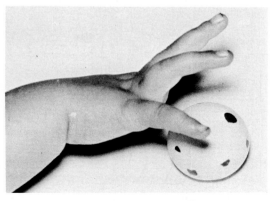

Fig. 6.18   Spastic hand with extreme extensor tone (from Illingworth R S 1987 The Development of the Infant and Young Child, 9th edn. Churchill Livingstone, Edinburgh).

nursery in the neonatal period and who were not walking independently at 18 months, 46% born before 28 weeks gestation were late walkers and at age 3, 56% had an associated abnormality. (This was cerebral palsy in a third of cases not all of whom had been diagnosed by 18 months (Johnson et al 1990).)

Shuffling and other prehensile forms of locomotion, including 'sitting-in-air' babies, are associated with late walking. A family history of late walking is relevant. There is a 50% incidence for heredity in late walkers (Hardie & MacFarlane 1980).

Faced with an 18-month-old child who is not yet walking, a careful perinatal and developmental milestone history and a detailed assessment of motor development and other developmental parameters is needed. Mental retardation or visual and/or auditory disabilities need excluding. Severe cerebral palsy will, hopefully, have been diagnosed by this age and the main differential diagnosis is between mild — or hypotonic — cases of cerebral palsy and Duchenne muscular dystrophy (rarely other congenital muscular dystrophies). Creatine phosphokinase is raised in Duchenne and possibly in the other dystrophies.

There is no agreement about the mean age of walking in Duchenne muscular dystrophy (Gardner-Medwin et al 1978). Unfortunately, many boys with Duchenne muscular dystrophy walk by 18 months (Crisp et al 1982) and so may not come to the attention of the developmentalist at this time. Children with cerebral palsy and mental retardation have delayed language and adaptive skills in addition to delayed motor development. The age for onset of language delay in Duchenne muscular dystrophy may be later. For example, in a study of 33 boys with Duchenne muscular dystrophy the mean age for language delay was 3.4 years (Smith et al 1990). Whether children with Duchenne dystrophy show delay in adaptive development at age 18 months is debatable; those whom I have seen have not had delayed adaptive development and I consider this a helpful differential diagnostic point, arguing against cerebral palsy with mental retardation, but this is not the experience of Illingworth (1987). Older children with Duchenne muscular dystrophy often show deficits such as poor mathematical ability and digit span which are believed to represent a deficit in short-term memory (Anderson et al 1988). The rarer forms of congenital muscular dystrophies are progressive and weakness in other muscles is found in addition to delayed walking.

Estimation of muscle tone is the best clinical tool in the differential diagnosis but can be extremely difficult. Two extremely useful discriminating signs of mild cases of cerebral palsy examined at this age are increased resistance to passive dorsiflexion at the ankle and cruising around furniture on the toes (Chaplais 1984). The former needs experience to assess and the DP should take every opportunity to estimate normal dorsiflexion by including it in his examination armamentarium. A method of testing for poor tone in the quadriceps is for the examiner to

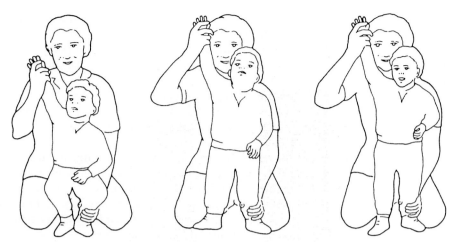

Fig. 6.19   Testing tone in quadriceps.

kneel on the floor with the child on his lap. One foot of the baby is placed firmly on the floor and held with the examiner's hand around the ankle. The DP pulls the baby's contralateral arm upwards and, if tone is good, the quadriceps contract (and can be felt to do so), the baby rising to the standing position. When tone is poor the arm is stretched but the baby flops forwards (Pollak & Fry 1986) (Fig. 6.19). Reflexes can be tested in this position; the tendon hammer coming from behind makes reflexes easy to elicit.

Delayed walking may occasionally be due to social causes.

Josie was admitted to hospital with a chest infection. A large $2\frac{1}{2}$-year-old she was not yet walking. Developmental assessment and examination uncovered no abnormality or delay. She could pull to stand, stand, but walk she would not. With physiotherapy help she was soon walking but not alone; she had to hold on to something, even someone's fifth finger. Whilst her paediatrician was thinking how to achieve her independence, Josie solved the problem herself. She walked along 'holding on' to her dress (Fig. 6.20). Josie was in unoffical fostercare and kept in her cot most of the day. Her story has a happy ending.

Ataxia

This term is confined to uncoordinated movements due to sensory or cerebellar lesions. Sensory lesions are usually worse in the absence of vision and affect the peripheral nerves or the posterior roots. Cerebellar lesions are unaffected by lack of visual guidance and are characterized by the absence of abnormal postural sensibility and movements tend to be jerky; nystagmus and dysarthria common. In Friedreich's (hereditofamilial) ataxia there is degeneration of spinocerebellar tracts so the ataxia is of the mixed type. A jerky ataxia is characteristic of the happy puppet syndrome of Angelman (Robb et al 1989).

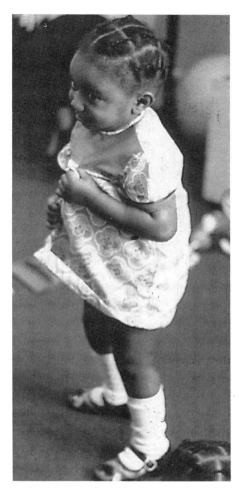

Fig. 6.20 Josie 'holding on' to her dress.

Cerebral palsy

Early diagnosis of *mild* cerebral palsy may be extremely difficult especially when there is no marked change in muscle tone. However there is always *delay in motor development* so it is essential to assess motor development in addition to a neurological examination. A full developmental examination in older children helps to distinguish mild cerebral palsy with normal mental development from mental retardation of unknown aetiology. In the latter, although mild motor delay may be present, the delay will be less than the delay in language and adaptive parameters. If delayed motor development is due to cerebral palsy it will eventually be accompanied by abnormal tone, posture and/or movements. The early diagnosis of cerebral palsy depends upon five factors:

- a suggestive history;
- persistence beyond normal time of some primitive reflexes especially the Moro, ATNR and the grasp reflex;
- delayed postural reactions such as head righting, the parachute (downward especially) and other postural corrections needed to maintain equilibrium (Fig. 6.21);
- paucity of movement. If a mother thinks that her baby does *not* use his limbs as much as expected she is usually correct but more commonly notices a difference between the two sides with hemiplegia the diagnosis;
- increased tone in some muscles may lead to clonus, equinus and exaggerated pronation.

The different types of cerebral palsy each have their own special feature, i.e. spastic and ataxic cerebral palsy being self-explanatory. Athetoid cerebral palsy displays involuntary movements with dystonia. Hemiplegic cerebral palsy is distinguished by differences on each side of the body. Not only is the diagnosis of cerebral palsy sometimes very difficult but the prognosis for eventual walking is also fraught with dangers (Holt 1981). The age of sitting may be the most helpful prognostic sign of the age of walking (Molnar 1979). The presence or absence of postural reflex has

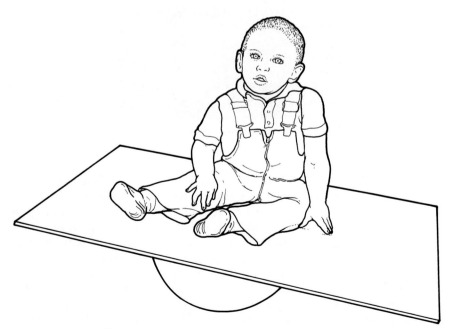

Fig. 6.21   Maintaining equilibrium, aged 10 months.

- When symptoms affect motor performance are both gross and fine motor development affected?
- How much does clumsiness affect general everyday life, schoolwork and/or social behaviour?
- Is the clumsiness making the parents and/or teachers and siblings irritated and hostile to the child, making him a scapegoat and sapping self-confidence?

Examination and diagnosis

If symptoms warrant further investigation, examination will include motor developmental status, measurement of visual acuity, personalsocial and language development, IQ and educational level in reading and spelling. The depth of the general medical examination depends upon an adverse history, the suspicion of muscular weakness or presence of a congenital lesion. Neurological examination is frequently necessary to exclude mild degrees of cerebral palsy, ataxia or, rarely, tumours.

The type of assessment will depend on answers to the following questions:

1. Is there developmental delay? If so, developmental status needs measuring.
2. Is abnormality present? If so it requires diagnosis.
3. Does a handicap with resultant dysfunction require estimation?
4. Is there a neurological basis to the problem?

Motor development will be assessed by tests described under normal development. The Stott test is recommended as the 'motor age' can be compared with norms for chronological age.

The handicap and dysfunction will be examined by methods described in Chapter 4.

Neurological basis will be examined either by a classical neurological examination or by paediatric modifications described by Touwen (1970) or Rutter et al (1970). Any child may need more than one type of examination. The proper assessment of a clumsy child takes a long time and is onerous for the child so a correct judgement as to which case to examine and which not is important.

Differential diagnosis

The differential diagnosis is between clumsiness, hyperactivity, mental retardation or brain damage (2, 3 or 4 may be present in the same child).

Differential diagnosis between clumsiness, hyperactivity and mental retardation

The young child

In 2–4-year-olds, the differential diagnosis can sometimes be made from the history and observation of hyperactivity but in 90% of cases both clumsy and hyperactive children are likely to be male so sex is not helpful in differential diagnosis. Clumsiness and hyperactivity may be associated with other evidence of neurodevelopmental delay such as late toilet training and expressive speech development whilst a history of general developmental delay is associated with mental retardation. A child determined to defy authority at all costs, be it his mother, parents or paediatrician, is probably an extreme example of the defiant, negative but essentially normal 2-year-old. On the other hand, a pleasantly mischievous child with a parent with no idea of authority or discipline who is completely at the child's mercy, probably has mother/child relationship problems which can be confirmed by finding difficulties at times when the two are together, e.g. mealtimes and bedtime.

When given constructional toys suitable for age, a hyperactive child will flit purposelessly from one toy to another using none appropriately and wander aimlessly around the room. A clumsy child will play appropriately but clumsily with the toys. An older mentally retarded child may behave like a hyperactive 2-4-year-old and the differential diagnosis between these two is the poor language development of the former.

The older child

The differential diagnosis in older children is less easy but hyperactive children move their bodies significantly more than normally active boys (Cammann et al 1989) and this will be observed during the history taking. Clumsiness may only affect specific movements. Hyperactivity is a sympton rather than a diagnosis and requires a differential diagnosis of its own (Schmidt et al 1987). Epidemiological surveys have found as many as one-third of all children have been described as overactive or distractible (Rutter et al 1970). It is salutary to consider the place in which hyperactivity is noted, as behaviour which teachers consider hyperactive might be considered in no way unusual in many homes and vice versa. Organized behaviour needs learning and practice neither of which may be forthcoming in some homes, with the result that children, unused to discipline or organization of their day, may give the appearance of hyperactivity. A child may not be hyperactive in the one-to-one setting such as the clinical setting yet is a total fidget sitting at the back of a large school class. Attention deficit is significantly more likely to be present in children with both 'reported' and 'clinically observable' hyperactivity (Leung 1988). Rutter et al (1970) described children as 'situationally' and 'pervasively' hyperactive. Schachar et al (1981) followed up these children four to five years later and found a distinct difference between the two types, the latter being strongly associated with disturbed behaviour, persistence of hyperactivity and impaired cognition. Boudreault et al (1988) distinguished between 'pervasive' and 'situational' attention deficit disorder (ADD). The pervasive ADDs had lower IQs and reading skills than situational ADDs who were more like non-ADDS in these skills. These findings alone justify a careful differential diagnosis of hyperactivity whenever it presents. The diagnosis of hyperactivity is 20 times more common in the US than in the UK (Taylor et al 1984). Prendergast et al (1988) report on an international study which interested readers are advised to read. The main reason for these large differences appears to be the fact that British clinicians diagnose conduct disorder in many children whom our American colleagues would label as the hyperkinetic syndrome or pervasive ADD.

Both clumsy and hyperactive children may have difficulties at school but there are differences which may help to separate them.

Clumsy children are likely to present with:

1. A history of developmental delay and abnormal proprioception (Johnston et al 1987)
2. A past history of executive speech delay.
3. Present articulation difficulty.
4. Specific learning problems, spelling and handwriting being more affected than reading.
5. Poor sport performance.
6. Asymmetry of the feet (Iloeje 1988).
7. A longer time in tapping tasks than normal controls (Schellekens et al 1983).

Hyperactive children on the other hand may have the following features:

1. Poor concentration and attention, both at home and school if of the pervasive type (Rapoport et al 1975).
2. Lack of shyness but may be antisocial.
3. Poor peer relations (Campbell & Paulaukas 1979).
4. Reading and spelling problems.
5. Lowered IQ especially if female (James & Taylor 1990).
6. Inability to exclude environmental distractions.
7. Inability to locate embedded figures (Hopkins et al 1979) — although Seci & Tishman (1984) do not agree.
8. A higher association with epilepsy and mental retardation than controls (Taylor 1986)

It may be necessary to undertake a modified neurological examination (Touwen et al 1970, Rutter et al 1970) to differentiate between the clumsiness and hyperactivity. Children with developmental *hyperactivity* are likely to have more clusters of 'soft' neurological signs, dyskinesia and associated movements than 'pure' *clumsy* children.

Degree of clumsiness

What is clumsiness? Taylor & McKinley (1979) conclude that children come to 'clumsiness' by a variety of routes which include lack of integrity of the central nervous system, slow maturity, inappropriate state of arousal and/or poor rehearsal. It is easier to differentiate between clumsiness and hyperactivity than it is to diagnose the *degree* of clumsiness. This is partly because the motor difficulty can range from a difficulty with spoon and fork and untidy writing to a severity making the formation of letters difficult, poor balance and gross motor abilities which label the patient a sport 'dunce'. Most *toddlers* are naturally very active, exploring hither and thither, but those of normal intelligence are purposeful in their curiosity and assessment of motor development at this age makes differential diagnosis between normal immature skills and real clumsiness extremely difficult, whilst that of hyperactivity is rather easier. Brand & Rosenbaum (1975) describe an observational method of recording children's movements which could be useful in recording clumsy movements and Rosenbloom & Horton (1970) presented a delightful method of measuring the degree of appropriate grasp, associated movements and proximal movements in young children. Clumsy 8-month-old babies explore and mouth objects less but show much visual observation (Kopp 1974).

By age 5, motor skills are developed enough to examine excessive clumsiness but children of this age do not normally have the gait nor some of the finer manipulative, sporting and athletic skills of adults. Previous inability to measure excessive clumsiness objectively has led many experts to question the validity of 'clumsiness' as a diagnosis. But there are now reliable methods for doing this.

Gubbay (1975) described a battery of 8 tests of motor proficiency for the diagnosis of developmental apraxia which he was able to condense to four tests all of which scored at or below the 5th percentile for children aged 6–12 years (Gubbay 1978). The Stott test (Henderson et al 1972) can be used for children aged 4–13 years and above. It is negatively scored with perfect performance having a score of 0, a failure in any of the five subsections a minus score of 2 and failure in every test at age level a minus score of 10. Tests for a lower age level add extra minus points. My clinical practice has been to consider children with a minus score of 10 as clumsy; minus 14 very clumsy and 18–20 as extremely clumsy.

PROGNOSIS OF MOTOR ABNORMALITIES

Changes in gross motor function are difficult to measure. Russell et al (1989) devised a gross motor function measure with videotape assessments which was found reliable in detecting change.

Cerebral palsy

Since cerebral palsy is a permanent but not progressive condition there is no cure or treatment as such but some symptoms and signs are likely to be less disabling than others. Athetoid cerebral palsy is less likely than other types to have associated mental retardation but more likely to have an associated deafness. Hemiplegia is usually the least severe type of cerebral palsy, many children leading almost normal lives. Cerebral palsies associated with other conditions such as mental retardation (approx. 50%) and convulsions (60%) have a poor prognosis (Hosking 1984). The mortality rate of the severely affected cerebral palsied is approximately 28 times that of an age and sex matched population, whilst a mild form has a three or four times higher rate. The death rate of males under 18 years of age with cerebral palsy is 13 times that of normal boys and for girls 17 times that of normal girls (Schlesinger et al 1959).

Clumsiness

Children with specific motor dyspraxia have a good prognosis, improving with time (Graham 1986). But they will rarely be amongst the winners of Olympic gold medals. When secondary problems of learning and lack of confidence are present improvement is less likely. Clumsy children followed up for three years continued to have more visuospatial problems than matched controls and were poor spellers with a high level of behaviour problems (Brenner et al 1967). A Swedish study that compared children at age 10 and 13 (Gillberg et al 1989) found their clumsiness was improved at the older age but school and behaviour problems continued in excess of matched controls. The children were not suffering specific dyspraxia but what the authors call 'damp', deficits in attention, motor control and perception.

Hyperactivity

By 14 years:

20% will be symptom free.
43% will be hyperactive with associated behavioural and learning problems.
37% will have behaviour and learning problems but not hyperactivity.

By 18 years:

81% will be symptom free.

In adolescence, hyperactive children are more likely than controls to show antisocial behaviour and substance abuse, have to repeat grades, be less good at maths and reading. Their outcome will *not* depend on: drug therapy, special education, psychological or motor therapy (Thorley 1988).

Outcome is related to IQ and socio-economic status and broken homes (Shaffer & Greenhill 1979).

MANAGEMENT

Management should only follow accurate diagnosis because the causes of motor delay or abnormality are varied and the treatment different for different aetiologies. It is becoming increasingly common for those whose gait needs studying in detail to visit a gait laboratory where sophisticated analysis can be carried out before deciding which treatment is required. This is partly because orthopaedic and surgical treatment have become increasingly sophisticated, partly because the fundamental divisions between operative and manipulative treatments are changing (Patrick 1989), and partly because the energy expended by the weight of any new equipment or surgical procedure can be calculated beforehand. In a child with motor delay there is sometimes a tendency to base treatment on the premise of 'walking at any cost'. Whether this is correct is debatable. The whole child must never be ignored at the expense of 'getting him walking'. His mental and social health merit equal consideration.

Management of cerebral palsy

The child's needs change with time and regular reassessments are necessary with the DP well placed to be the conductor of the team that will inevitably be involved in treatment. Orthopaedic surveillance is needed to ensure that hips do not dislocate, joints do not contract and spastic muscles do not shorten. The difficulty of early diagnosis in many cases of cerebral palsy has been mentioned with motor delay as the only sign. This has implications for treatment. Should one attempt to treat motor delay per se so babies who later are shown to suffer cerebral palsy have received early treatment? Most DPs will have to decide their stance on this question, a decision not made any easier by the ambiguous views on the effects of early treatment. Physical maturation is slower in children with cerebral palsy so motor milestones will be late although most eventually improve, especially walking and in diplegics (Patrick 1989). There is a case for the use of physiotherapy and occupational therapy up to the age of 7 years and reserving surgery for older age groups.

Physiotherapy

There are several schools of thought on the objectives, types and results of physiotherapy. Present-day physiotherapy treatment is very much more than the passive stretching of muscles and, particularly amongst those practising the Bobath method (Bobath & Bobath 1964), involves the active participation of the child. It has much to offer in giving a sense of normal movement, particularly to the young palsied baby and toddler. The mother and her palsied child are seeing the physiotherapist on a regular basis and she/he will be the recipient of many of the mother's fears and anxieties; most experienced physiotherapists are excellent carers, providing psychological support to the accompanying parent. They are also monitors of the marital and home situation and can alert the paediatrician to any problems. I consider their role in the care of the young cerebral palsied invaluable. Whether they are best qualified for this counselling role is debatable but, in clinical practice, often more is revealed whilst the mother sits beside her child having his treatment than in the 'artificial' situation of a counselling session. Not all will agree with this view.

There has been a considerable upsurge of interest in and parental pressure for the introduction of the system of conductive education as practised at the Peto Institute in Budapest. For a balanced and thoughtful critique readers are recommended to read Robinson et al (1989). One of the concerns of the Peto system is whether the 'Conductor' can be 'everything' to the child over long stretches of time. This contrasts with the situation in the UK, in which many children receive uncoordinated help from a variety of therapists, often in different places. A middle view is that taken by well-integrated child development centres (see Ch. 15).

Biofeedback training

Biofeedback has been suggested to suppress abnormal muscle contractions by electromyogram signals with accompanying teaching programmes. Nash et al (1989) report reduced spasticity in gastrocnemius muscle in children as young as 4 years by such a method. It was inexpensive and had the advantage that it was presented as a video game. Tardieu et al (1984) believe that some cerebral palsied children might be helped by improving their awareness of proprioceptive signals from muscle contractions and joints.

Orthopaedic treatment

Splints and plaster casting aim to promote muscle growth and prevent contractures by the lengthening of muscle. These measures are often successful but not if the increase in length over which the muscle can contract is offset by increased spasm.

Motorized wheelchairs can be successfully used by children as young as 20 months (Butler 1983).

Surgical treatment American surgeons have led the way to more sophisticated surgical treatment of posture and walking deformities. They have based surgery on dynamics after full analysis of gait. The 'Birthday syndrome' in which children remember their birthdays by their operations beginning at age 7 has been described (Patrick 1989).

Management of Duchenne muscular dystrophy

Physiotherapy in the ambulant stage may prevent contractures but the inevitable deterioration will progress to a wheelchair existence. Learning problems and a lowering of intelligence are common, schooling becomes extremely difficult if not impossible and it may be advisable to opt for private tutoring at an early rather than late stage. The children may become obese and require to diet and there is a need to be alert to cardiac symptoms. Management is of the whole child and his family.

Management of clumsiness

Just as the diagnosis of clumsiness and hyperactivity is a contentious issue so too is treatment. Many consider that no treatment is indicated and the evidence is that clumsiness improves with time. Physiotherapy and occupational therapy programmes are often prescribed. These range from treating individual faults or delays to general gymnastic programmes and may be intensive over a short time or weekly over longer periods. A programme at King's College Hospital consisted of weekly sessions. The children were given individual physiotherapy work on items of the Stott assessment which they were failing. This was followed by 10 minutes of general gymnasium play with other children. A course lasted 5 months. 90% improved their Stott scores when reassessed. However there were no controls and all the children had reading, spelling and/or writing difficulties which did not show any improvement. 'Clumsy' children are used to physical failure and are timid, socially gauche and often the butt of the family. One aspect of the programme was the obvious improvement in the children's self-confidence, which had the effect that they were not so irritating to other family members and this unquantifiable item was probably the main gain of the programme and could have been acquired by other means.

If clumsy children are assessed using the Stott programme, the vast majority of them have problems of gross motor movement and balance and it is rare to find a child who is clumsy only in fine manipulation. A programme was carried out in the Scottish Rite Children's Hospital, Dallas (unpublished) which, apart from work on the children's individual failures, concluded with a group rhythm-with-music class. Whether the children improved was not scientifically recorded but the attempts made by the children to dance and make rhythmic movements showed how handicapped these children are.

Management of hyperactivity

There is no evidence that intolerance of *food additives* is a major cause of hyperactivity (Taylor 1986). It is not general practice in the UK, therefore, to prescribe special diets as treatment. The use of *drugs* in hyperactivity is also uncertain although many in the US claim good results. Stimulants are the drugs of choice.

REFERENCES

Ainsworth M 1967 Infancy in Uganda, 73. Johns Hopkins Press, Baltimore

Amiel-Tison C 1980 Possible acceleration of neurological maturation following high-risk pregnancy. American Journal of Obstetrics and Gynecology 138: 303–306

Anderson S W, Routh D K, Ionasescu V V 1988 Serial position memory of boys with Duchenne muscular dystrophy. Developmental Medicine and Child Neurology 30: 328–333

Annett M 1985 Left, right, hand and brain: the right shift theory. Erlbaum, London

Batheja M, McManus I C 1985 Handedness in the mentally handicapped. Developmental Medicine and Child Neurology 27: 63–68

Bax M 1980 Editorial. Left hand, right hand. Developmental Medicine and Child Neurology 22: 567–568

Berges J, Lezine I 1965 The imitation of gestures. Clinics in Developmental Medicine 18. Spastics International Medical Publications/Heinemann Medical Books, London

Bishop D V M 1980 Handedness, clumsiness and cognitive ability. Developmental Medicine and Child Neurology 22: 569–579

Bleck E E 1971 The shoeing of children: sham or science? Developmental Medicine and Child Neurology 13: 188–195

Bleck E E 1975 Locomotor prognosis in cerebral palsy. Developmental Medicine and Child Neurology 17: 18–25

Bobath K, Bobath B 1964 The facilitation of normal postural reactions and movements in the treatment of cerebral palsy. Physiotherapy 50: 3

Bottos M, Barba B D, Stefani D, Pettena G, Tonin C, D'Este A 1989 Locomotor strategies preceding independent walking: prospective study of neurological and language development in 424 cases. Developmental Medicine and Child Neurology 31: 25–34

Boudreault M, Thivierge J, Cote R, Boutin P, Julien Y, Bergeron S 1988 Cognitive development and reading achievement in pervasive-ADD, situational-ADD and control children. Journal of Child Psychology and Psychiatry and Allied Disciplines 29: 611–619

Brand H L, Rosenbaum P 1975 Recording children's movements: the development of an observational method. In: Holt K S (ed) Movement and Child Development. Clinics in Developmental Medicine 55. Spastics International Medical Publication/Heinemann Medical Books, London

Brenner W M, Gillman S, Zangwill O, Farrell M 1967 Visuo-motor disability in school children. British Medical Journal 4: 259–262

British Medical Journal 1981 Leading article. Left hand, right hand. 1: 588

Brown J K, von Rensburg F, Walsh G, Lakie M, Wright G W 1987 A neurological study of hand function of hemiplegic children. Developmental Medicine and Child Neurology 29: 287–304

Bruininks R H 1978 The Bruininks–Oseretsky Test of Motor Proficiency. NFER–Nelson, Windsor

Butler C, Okamoto G A, McKay T M 1983 Powered mobility for very young disabled children. Developmental Medicine and Child Neurology 254: 472–474

Butler P, Engelbrecht M, Major R E, Tait J H, Stallard J, Patrick J H 1984 Physiological cost index of walking for normal children and its use as an indicator of physical handicap. Developmental Medicine and Child Neurology 26: 607–612

Cammann R, Miehlke A 1989 Differentiation of motor activity of normally active and hyperactive boys in schools: some preliminary results. Journal of Child Psychology and Psychiatry and Allied Disciplines 30.6: 899–906

Campbell S B, Paulaukas S 1979 Peer relations in hyperactive children. Journal of Child Psychology and Psychiatry and Allied Disciplines 20: 233–246

Capute A J, Shapiro B K, Palmer F B, Ross A, Wachtel R C 1985 Normal gross motor development: the influences of race, sex and socio-economic status. Developmental Medicine and Child Neurology 27: 635–643

Castner B M 1939 Handedness and eyedness of children referred to a guidance clinic. Psychological Research 3: 99–112

Cech D, Gallagher R J, Josephs A, Pearl O 1983 Assessment of motor abilities of infants, using the Chicago Infant Neuromotor Assessment. University of Chicago, Illinois

Chaplais J de Z 1984 The late walking child. In: Macfarlane J A (ed) Progress in child health, vol 1, Churchill Livingstone, Edinburgh

Cratty B J, Martin M M 1969 Perceptual-motor efficiency in children. Lea & Febiger, Philadelphia

Crisp D E, Ziter F A, Bray P F 1982 Diagnostic delay in Duchenne's muscular dystrophy. Journal of the American Medical Association 247: 478–480

Crome L C, Stern J 1967 Pathology of mental retardation. Churchill, Livingstone, Edinburgh

Crouchman M 1986 The effects of babywalkers on early locomotor development. Developmental Medicine and Child Neurology 28: 757–761

Curti M, Marshall F B, Steggerda M 1935 The Gesell schedules applied to 1-, 2- and 3-year-old negro children of Jamaica. Journal of Comparative Psychology 20: 125

de Chateau P, Andersson Y 1976 Left-side preference for holding and carrying newborn infants. II. Doll-holding and carrying from 2 to 16 years. Developmental Medicine and Child Neurology 18: 738–744

Donoghue E C, Kirman B H, Bullmore G H L, Labanm D, Abbas K A 1970 Some factors affecting age of walking in a mentally retarded population. Developmental Medicine and Child Neurology 12: 781–792

Dubowitz V, Hersov L 1976 Management of children with non-organic (hysterical) disorders of motor function. Developmental Medical and Child Neurology 18: 358–368

Egan D F, Illingworth R S, MacKeith R C 1969 Developmental screening 0–5 years. Clinics in Developmental Medicine 30. Spastics International Medical Publications/Heinemann Medical Books, London

Elliott J M, Connolly K J 1984 A classification of manipulative hand movements. Developmental Medicine and Child Neurology 26: 283–296

Elliott J M, Connolly K J, Doyle A J R 1988 Development of kinaesthetic sensitivity and motor performance in children. Developmental Medicine and Child Neurology 30: 80–92

English school children: a questionnaire survey. Journal of Abnormal Child Psychology 12: 143–156

Frankenburg W K, Dodds J B 1967 The Denver Developmental Screening Test. Journal of Pediatrics 71: 181

Gardner-Medwin D, Bundey S, Green S 1978 Early diagnosis of Duchenne muscular dystrophy. Lancet i: 1102

Geber M, Dean R F 1957 Gesell tests on African children. Pediatrics 20: 1055

Geber M, Dean R F 1964 Le developpement psychomoteur et somatique des jeunes enfants Africains en Ouganda. Courrier 14: 425

Gesell A 1933 The mental growth of prematurely born infants. Journal of Pediatrics 2: 676–680

Gesell A, Amatruda C S 1947 Developmental diagnosis. Hoeber, New York

Gesell A, Amatruda C S, Ames L B et al 1966 The first five years of life. Methuen, London

Gesell A, Ames L B 1947 The development of handedness. Journal of General Psychology 70: 155–175

Gillberg C, Rasmussen P, Carlstrom G, Svenson B, Waldenstrom E 1982 Perceptual, motor, attentional deficits in six-year-old children: epidemiological aspects. Journal of Child Psychology and Psychiatry and Allied Disciplines 23.2: 131–144

Gillberg I C, Gillberg C 1989 Children with preschool minor neurodevelopmental disorders. IV. Behaviour and school achievement at age 13. Developmental Medicine and Child Neurology 31: 3–13

Graffar M, Corbier J 1972 Contribution to the study of the influence of socio-economic conditions on the growth and development of the child. Early Child Development and Care 1: 141–179

Graham P 1986 Child psychiatry: a developmental approach. Oxford Medical, Oxford

Grant W W, Boelsche A, Zin D 1973 Developmental patterns of two motor functions. Developmental Medicine and Child Neurology 15: 171–177

Tew B 1979 Differences between Welsh and Canadian children on parts of the Test of Motor Impairment. Child: Care, Health and Development 5: 135–141

Thelen E, Cooke D W 1987 Relationship between newborn stepping and later walking: a new interpretation. Developmental Medicine and Child Neurology 29: 380–393

Thorley G 1988 Adolescent outcome for hyperactive children. Archives of Disease in Childhood 63: 1181–1183

Touwen B C L 1971 A study of the development of some motor phenomena in infancy. Developmental Medicine and Child Neurology 13: 435

Touwen B C L 1976 The neurological development in Infancy. Clinics in Developmental Medicine 58. Spastics International Medical Publications/Heinemann Medical Books, London

Touwen B C L, Prechtl H 1970 The neurological examination of the child with minor nervous dysfunction. Clinics in Developmental Medicine 38. Spastics International Medical Publications/Heinemann Medical Books, London

Waters R L, Hislop H J, Thomas L, Campbell J 1983 Energy cost of walking in normal children and teenagers. Developmental Medicine and Child Neurology 25: 184–188

Weggemann T, Brown J K, Fulford G E, Minns R A 1987 A study of normal baby movements. Child: Care, Health and Development 13: 41–58

Wiegersma P H, van der Velde A 1983 Motor development of deaf children. Journal of Child Psychology and Psychiatry and Allied Disciplines 24: 103–111

Willemse J 1986 Benign idiopathic dystonia with onset in the first year of life. Developmental Medicine and Child Neurology 28: 355–363

Williams L O, Anderson A D, Campbell J, Thomas L, Feiwell E, Walker J M 1983 Energy cost of walking and of wheelchair propulsion by children with myelodysplasia: comparison with normal children. Developmental Medicine and Child Neurology 25: 617–624

Wolff P H, Gunnoe C E, Cohen C 1983 Associated movements as a measure of developmental age. Developmental Medicine and Child Neurology 25: 417–429

Wyke B 1975 The neurological basis of movement – a developmental review. In: Holt K (ed) Movement and child development. Clinics in Developmental Medicine 55. Spastics International Medical Publications/Heinemann Medical Books, London

Zdanska-Brincken M, Wolanski N 1969 A graphic method for the evaluation of motor development in infants. Developmental Medicine and Child Neurology 11: 228–241

Ziviani J 1983 Qualitative changes in dynamic tripod grip between seven and 14 years of age. Developmental Medicine and Child Neurology 25: 778–782

height at *15 months*; he is physically active and dislikes dressing. *By 18 months* he take off pants, shoes, socks and can undo easy zips and big buttons. *By 3 years* he begins to dress and likes to attempt dressing alone. *At 4 years* clothes are rarely back to front and both sexes enjoy dressing up. Most children can dress and undress themselves by *5 years* except for shoelaces, small and back buttons; they like to choose their clothes but are uninterested in their care. *By 6 years* dressing is personal habit, some being very interested in their clothes and others not. Some girls are interested in hairstyles. *By 7 years* most children choose their own clothes.

These developmental stages are those which may be considered as Western standards. In many areas of the world with hot climates and several-generation-families quite different routines are found. However, 15 different ethnic groups of 300+ 3-year-olds around the world showed a remarkable similarity in eating, sleeping, dressing and sphincter control. West Indian, American Negro and Ethiopean immigrants to Israel were less advanced in sphincter control but more independent in eating, dressing and going to bed. Bedouins (living a nomadic life in the Negev desert) and Vietnamese 'boat' children (living in a transit camp in Hong-Kong) were more independent in most skills compared with Caucasians (Pollak 1988).

DEVELOPMENT OF PERSONALITY

Personality is that aspect of a person which is unique to the individual, but there is no agreement on definition so it is impossible to describe development of personality, although there is no doubt that development takes place and that babies are different from birth. There is no lack of theories of behaviour. The learning theorists conceive behaviour as the result of reinforcement of a behavioural pattern (e.g. Bandura 1977). The ethological view is of prepatterned signals and responses (e.g. Lorenz 1966, Bowlby 1951); the psychoanalytical notion is of instinctive drives inducing behaviour. Personality has basic structures which engage in activities for the gratification of these basic instincts (e.g. Freud 1960, Erikson 1963). A difference between Freud and Erikson is that the former describes psychosexual phases and the latter psychosocial phases.

There are biological theories. Body build has been associated with personality types (Sheldon 1940); Freedman (1979) has described differences of responses of newborn babies in different ethnic groups, whilst Buss et al (1975) have described four temperamental dimensions which they consider to be inherited. The developmentalist can safely accept multifactorial influence, since personality is extremely complex, and take from each theory what seems appropriate to clinical observation and practice. For example, the learning theory sees a pattern of behaviour as the result of the reinforcement of that behaviour. If true, the reinforcement (probably the environment) can be subjected to change and practical therapy applied to obtain changes in behaviour.

Emotional development

Emotions are described as changes in arousal levels (Darwin 1872) accompanied by physiological changes such as alterations in heart or respiratory rate; are difficult to measure; subject to developmental change and helped to maturity by developmental changes in other parameters such as higher cognitive skills, increased attention spans, reasoning skills and increased social experiences. There is increasing differentiation. Changes lead to increasing degrees of self-help and social adeptness leads to understanding feelings in others and learning to wait for gratification. Autistic and anxious-depressed children are less efficient than normal children in recognizing emotion in facial expressions (Walker 1981). Some emotions which undergo development are: crying, smiling and laughing, anxiety, jealousy, anger and aggression.

Crying

A newborn cries about two hours a day (Gesell et al 1946). Babies who 'room-in' with their mothers cry less than those who are in a communal nursery. Crying — a baby's most eloquent expression — is a response to hunger or pain but other provoking factors may be temperature and undressing (Wolff 1969), coverings and examination (Bayley 1932). *By 24 weeks* a baby cries from frustration and loud noises and at *36 weeks* to gain

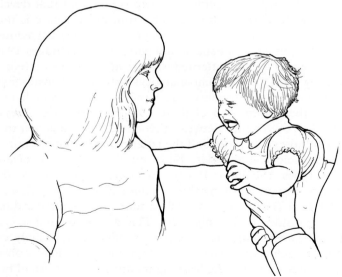

Fig. 7.4   Crying for 'mummy'.

usually towards a younger sibling. But *7 years* is the height of jealousy; girls are jealous of a father's attention to their mother but both sexes show jealousies towards siblings, imagining parental favouritism. They are jealous of possessions and unwilling to share. Use of the Bene/Anthony Family relations test reveals a surprisingly high incidence of jealousy but whether this is justified or only the child's assumption is not possible to assess.

Anger and aggression

Babies are said not to display anger or aggression until towards the *end of the first year* (Helms & Turner 1976) although when one listens to the cry of some younger babies one could imagine they are angry. The first anger may be brought on by frustration such as the casting of a toy which disappears without recovery (Gesell et al 1946). Aggressive acts are most common during the *second and third years* (Goodenough 1931) (Fig. 7.8) when they are part of the 'terrible twos'. Screaming, kicking and sometimes biting, with temper tantrums are common. At first acts of aggression are directed towards adults, particularly the main caregiver, but later are directed towards other children. These initial acts are only aggressive acts with non-aggressive ends in mind (Schaffer 1985). *15-month-olds* do not usually look at each other but only at the toy they want to grab (Bronson

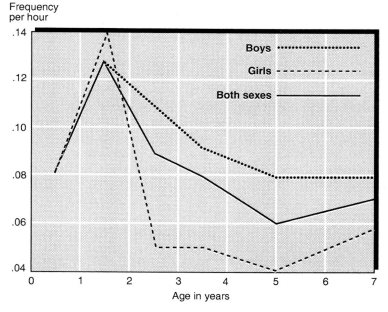

Fig. 7.8   Frequency of anger outbursts (From Goodenough F L 1931 Anger in Young Children. Minnesota Press, Minneapolis. Courtesy of the University of Minnesota).

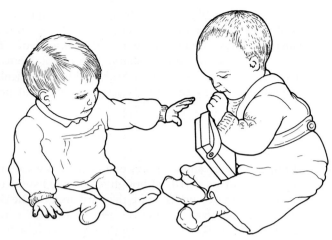

Fig. 7.9   Only looking at the toy, aged 15 months.

1975) (Fig. 7.9). *After 3 years* children are becoming both physically and verbally aggressive towards each other ('That's mine!' 'Mandy have it!' 'Me want!'). Gradually, aggression is less physical and more verbally abusive and threatening ('I hate you!' 'I'll kill you!') until *6–7 years* when boys in particular become physically aggressive towards play- and schoolmates, usually about possessions. Physical aggression is also matched by verbal threats. By *8–9 years* most physical aggression has faded although still part of boy's rough and tumble play.

Several factors affect aggression:

Sex. Boys are physically more aggressive than girls at all ages (Maccoby et al 1974, 1980) and four times more likely to show aggressive antisocial behaviour (Rutter 1970). Gang warfare is a predominantly male pursuit as is football hooliganism. There is insufficient evidence to associate aggression with Y chromosomes or Androgen levels (Shaffer & Johnson 1980).

Parental behaviour. Parents who are inconsistent but violent in dealing out punishment have more aggressive children (Delaney 1965). Rejecting and cold parents also tend to have more aggressive children (Gordon & Smith 1980). A combination of these factors, especially in fathers, increases the likelihood of aggression in their children (Sears et al 1957, Rutter et al 1970).

Social class. Both pre- and school-age children from lower socio-economic classes show more aggression than those from higher social classes (Goldstein 1955, Glueck & Glueck 1962). When combined with the type of parenting outlined above, the effects are compounded (Martin 1975).

Culture. Some ethnic groups are traditionally nonaggressive such as the Pygmies in Central Africa and the Arapesh in New Guinea, whilst others, e.g. the Il tribe in Uganda and the Mundugumor in New Guinea

(Turnbull 1972) have highly aggressive societies. Their children tend to take after their parents.

Learning that aggression pays. Children learn from parents (Jersild & Markey 1935), teachers (Bandura 1961) or television (Eron et al 1972). Aggressive behaviour is more likely to occur during a high arousal state and after situations in which violence has been seen to pay.

Other factors. Children with low IQs, and some handicaps (e.g. Asperger' syndrome) show an increased tendency towards aggression and, when combined with other factors such as social class and/or parental attitudes, this tendency is compounded. Inexperience with alcohol ingestion causes aggression in some adolescents (Pollak 1989).

Aggression in any child remains surprisingly constant during the childhood years. Two studies (Olweus 1978, Lowenstein 1978) of bullies and boys who had been bullied concluded that bullies are more likely to have positive attitudes to aggression whilst the bullied boys were more likely to be anxious. Both suggest that the boys who were bullied benefit from social skills training (see below).

The development of self and sexual identity

Self

Newborns probably do not have a concept of themselves but Piaget believes that a *one-month-old* baby is aware of some bodily movements and gradually learns the limits of his body. By *6 months* he learns both to transfer an object from one hand to another hand and that his body has two parts which meet in the middle. By *4–8 months*, by repeating actions external to himself (e.g. waving a rattle), he learns that objects exist outside of himself. Children become aware of themselves as a separate person at *18 months* in a development which is thought to be social rather than cognitive, as mentally retarded children (Hill & Tomlin 1981) and monkeys (Gallup 1979) develop the concept about the same time as normally intelligent humans. *2-year-olds* identify a photograph of themselves and by *3 years* can say 'me, I,' even 'mine' and learn to distinguish between others, e.g. they recognize a person is a stranger. By *age 4* they recognize a doll or inanimate object cannot think (Maccoby 1980). *By 8 years* children make subjective and accurate judgements about themselves and their peers (Harter 1982). Adolescents lose self-esteem in their teens in an 'identity crisis' (Shaffer 1985). There has been little research into the development of self identity of handicapped children but the most vulnerable period appears to be adolescence (Graham 1986). Some with obvious physical defects have a low self-esteem which begins when sports are important and some children with cerebral palsy have visuo-spatial problems (see Ch. 13), and show by their drawings that they have problems in concepts of their body shape.

Sexual identity

Physical identification of sex begins with the chromosomal differences of the fetus. Males secrete testosterone during the gestational period whilst females do not secrete any sex hormone. Sex hormones secrete only in late childhood in both sexes and puberty occurs around 12–14 years. *3–3½-year-olds* probably know their own sex and recognize that of others. Permanence of gender is recognized at *4–7 years*. Children of different sexes are treated differently from earliest babyhood but whether this accounts for differences in attitudes between sexes is extremely doubtful. By *nursery school age* there is a tendency for sex-typed activities to have become established, boys earlier than girls and by *school age* children choose their own sex both to play with and as friends. An examination of bedrooms at this age will easily identify the sex of the occupant! Lower social compared with middle-class children are more sex-typed (Morgan 1982) but this may be changing.

The development of morality

Piaget (1932) is the developmentalist who has written most widely on this subject and sees morality as learning and understanding the need for rules in society. Until 5 years of age children are thought to be 'amoral' but learn (from older children and adults) some rules of games and life which they believe are inviolate. The next stage is 'moral realism' when children judge whether an action is right or wrong by the harm which ensues and later children can intellectually moralize. Piaget's theories have been challenged by others. In view of the importance of morality for social harmony and justice, it is surprising that not more attention is given to the teaching of it in schools. Lynn (1988) has pointed out that it is in the curriculum of every Japanese school.

SOCIAL DEVELOPMENT

The way a baby learns to 'bond' or 'attach' to one person has been the subject of intense research (Bowlby 1958, 1969, Maccoby & Masters 1970, Schaffer & Emerson 1964, Schaffer 1971, Ainsworth 1973, Rutter 1972). Their major findings are well known and need no repeating. The attachment or bonding of a baby to an adult is subject to phases of development.

Phases of attachment

As auditory and visual perceptive skills begin to mature, commonly occurring phenomena such as mother's voice and form are gradually distinguished by the developing baby. Babies can distinguish their mother's voice from a stranger's and develop a preference for looking at the human face. But they are not passive in these observations and react by smiling, crying and touching (Rutter 1980) and physiologically with increased heart rate and dilation of the pupils. Their mothers also react to them (Minde 1986). Thus begins a two-way process and the baby's first social reactions; that this early intimate contact and interaction between mother and baby reaps rewards in promoting love between both has been amply demonstrated (Klaus et al 1970, 1972, Klaus & Kennell 1976, Kennell 1974, Gomes-Pedro et al 1984).

By 6 months the strong attachment enters a selective phase and develops between baby and mother. In addition to learning to distinguish between strangers and parents, babies develop an attachment to their mother, dislike being separated from her and become wary of strangers. Their first 'love affair' has begun. The ability to reach out and want to be picked up coincides with an intense clinging to their major caregiver. This reaction occurs in many different cultures (Ainsworth 1967, Rutter 1980) and many animals (Bowlby 1967). As in all social encounters, these responses depend not only on the child but also his environment (and caregiver). The bonding of a baby to his first adult is one of the finest examples of social behaviour requiring the participation of both persons to be satisfactory. Around *18 months* there follows what Rutter (1980) graphically describes as the 'secure base effect'. Because the child has formed an attachment to his main caregiver he feels secure. This stage is reached just as he is becoming mobile and interested in an environment wider than his mother's immediate presence; is learning to talk and is more aware of others (including pets). Thus all developmental parameters conspire to encourage the child to widen his attachment to others in the family and/or other caregivers and the stage of *social attachments* begins. The child learns increasingly to separate from his 'deep' attachment. He can understand object permanence, has some concept of time and so can believe that what is not seen may not necessarily be gone for ever, which allows him to move further away into the presence of strangers, adult and child, without suffering anxiety. He knows his mother still exists even if he cannot see her. When a secure attachment is formed, personalsocial and language development are enhanced (Main et al 1985). Before social attachments can be formed, however, the child needs language with which to communicate and to have enough understanding of role playing to 'give and take' and delayed social development is often seen in language-delayed children.

Social attachments can be divided into those with adults and with children. The characteristics of these attachments overlap but there is evidence to show that they are different (Maccoby 1980).

Social attachments between children

Children behave differently towards their elders or juniors than towards their peers. Children of both sexes, several years older than their siblings,

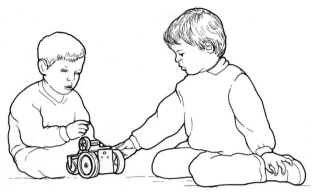

Fig. 7.10   Jealous of toy.

are likely to assume a protective role towards younger children but, when the age difference is less, an assertive role is more common, the younger child usually accepting a compliant and dependent role (Whiting & Whiting 1970). Children interacting with children of the same age are more likely to be sociable to each other. Despite wide personal differences some developmental patterns can be seen between children of similar ages. At *1 year* children of similar ages have an alternating pattern of attraction and rejection and interest in the presence of other children is object (toy!) related (Fig. 7.10). By *2 years* real social exchange occurs; children imitate each other and enact give-and-take roles. They play in twos even in the presence of many others and aggressive acts are seen as well as friendly ones. Piaget (1926) described children's thoughts as egocentric, seeing everything from their own perspective and believed that only when the 'concrete thought' stage was reached (around 7 years of age) could children understand the views of others, but Hobson (1980) has successfully challenged this view. By *3–4 years* there is interchild interaction by talking, playing and crying. At *4–6 years* children have more elaborate social intercourse and can cope with bigger groups. Same-sex grouping is beginning. From *6 years* group or team social interaction increases but also so do 'best' friendships.

Groups and teams

Initially, children do not understand common aims well and social behaviour in groups is individualistic and less cooperative than it later becomes. There is increasing cooperation with time and children are able to ask the opinions of individuals. 'Social rules' are learnt and children play team games, able to understand the needs of a team as opposed to those of the whole group and are now secure with their peers. In adolescence, cliques or gangs, more common amongst boys than girls, are formed. Initially unisex, an element of heterosexuality is later introduced during the teens.

When dating starts the cliques begin to disintegrate and couples become attached to each other (Dunphy 1963).

Friendships

At *6–8 years* children are drawn to each other through frequent meetings and sharing activities. Usually of the same sex, boys tend to have more friends than girls, whose smaller circle is possibly more intense (Hartup 1980). At *8–10 years* children choose friends who have the same values because of shared interests. At *10–14 years* real friendships, based not only upon shared interests and values but involving a real understanding of the needs of the other, are formed. Children are able to confide in each other. In the case of children with poor family relationships this ability to confide in others can be extremely important (Pollak 1979).

Attachments to adults

Children as young as 14–24 months of age have different attachments to adults as with other children. They differ in behaviour towards their mothers and adult strangers, being more likely to interact with the former by smiling, talking and touching. They are more likely to respond to other children than to strange adults and, in the presence of a strange adult, cry and are more aggressive towards other children. As children become older they tolerate strange adults better, assimilating them by the presence of their mother until they are able to separate happily (Rheingold & Eckerman 1975). Children enjoy rough-and-tumble play with each other but rarely enter into this play with adults to whom their reaction is likely to be one of compliance, dependence and attention-seeking and they petition adults rather than children. Adults' and children's worlds overlap, and parents exercise influence on relations with peers by their provision of opportunities to meet other children, both by choice of school and neighbourhood play. Whether it is necessary for children to have a satisfactory relationship with their parents to give them the trust and security that allows them to socialize with their peers is discussed later.

Attachments to inanimate objects

Winnicott (1954) believed that attachment to inanimate objects such as cuddly toys is an important developmental stage, representing transition between inner and external reality. Having an attachment object at 3 years is more common amongst children who are considered to be independent. Thumb sucking or sucking other objects is related to attachment to an inanimate object (Boniface & Graham 1979) and, at this age, may have a substitution function.

FACTORS WHICH AFFECT PERSONALSOCIAL DEVELOPMENT

These might be divided into the following:

- Factors in the child.
- Effects of parents and home.
- Environmental factors.

Factors in the child

Position in family

If the baby is unwanted or the youngest in a large family there may be difficulty in bonding (Shaffer 1985) with subsequent behaviour problems (Davie et al 1972).

Temperament

Neonates differ in irritability and alertness (Brazelton 1979). The 'slow-to-warm-up' baby has been described as has the 'difficult' baby (Thomas & Chess 1977); these temperamental dispositions remain constant throughout childhood (Sigvardsson et al 1987). Some parents have difficulty in establishing good social interactions with both types of babies (Greene et al 1983). The 'slow-to-warm-up' babies have a predisposition to develop withdrawal and anxiety feelings leading to a lack of exploring strange situations (Graham 1986, Batter & Davidson 1979, Dunn et al 1981) whilst 'difficult' babies are associated with behavioural and conduct disorders (Graham et al 1973). The importance of personal characteristics and temperament to the outcome of 'coping' or not with stress has been noted (Rutter 1981).

Physical conditions

Maturation. Maturational age may affect children's personalsocial development since early adolescent maturers are, on average, superior to late maturers on achievement and mental ability tests (Westin-Lingren 1982). Late maturation is associated with enuresis (Shaffer et al 1984, Oppel et al 1968) and thus, at 7 years of age, with clumsiness, speech defects, perceptual dysfunction (Jarvelin 1989), all of which are expressions of late neurodevelopmental maturity.

Pre-term babies. These babies are less active and responsive, vocalizing and smiling less than fullterm babies and averting gaze and bodies more frequently and generally showing a less positive affect (Crnic et al 1983) all of which affect social development. Prematurity alone is no longer associated with bonding problems but child abuse is associated with both and physically abused children show personalsocial abnormalities of development (Oates 1984).

and inaccurate. However, there is no doubting that behaviour problems, particularly in the preschool child, are common. For example, 83% of a sample of health visitors reported behaviour problems as the major part of their caseload (Hewitt et al 1989).

Children under 3.5 years

Ghodsian et al (1988) studied mild behaviour problems in one of the poorer London boroughs. The prevalence rate was:

7% at 0–4 months
43% at 5–6 months
21% between 7–9 months
29% between 10–15 months

Hart et al (1984) studied mild personalsocial behavioural problems and found the following prevalence rates:

Night waking
11% at 2 years
16% at 3 years
9.5% at $4\frac{1}{2}$ years

Poor appetite
21% at 1 year
17% at 18 months
12% at 3 years
10% at $4\frac{1}{2}$ years

Temper tantrums
19% of 2-year-olds had 1+ daily tantrum
18% of 3-year-olds
11% of $4\frac{1}{2}$ year olds

Difficulties in management
5% of 2-year-olds
8% of 3-year-olds
7% of $4\frac{1}{2}$-year-olds

In a London borough the rate of behaviour and emotional disorder of 3-year-olds was: 7% had a moderate or severe behavioural problem and 15% had mild behaviour problems (Richman et al 1975). *No* social class differences were found nor was the rate higher amongst West Indian children (Earls & Richman 1980). The disturbed children were associated with poor quality of marital relationship, maternal depression and social deprivation. 63% of the children had continuing problems at 4 years of age. Boys differed from girls both in frequency and symptomatology

(Richman et al 1982). Similar findings were reported in preschool children in Newcastle (Miller et al 1960) and in the USA (Minde & Minde 1977).

Jenkins et al (1980) and Bax & Hart (1976) studied the same behavioural symptoms and noted changes in prevalence rates between 2 and $4\frac{1}{2}$ years of age, behavioural symptoms being more common at age 3 than at age 2 with improvement in all symptoms, except dependency, by $4\frac{1}{2}$ years.

Children of school age

Psychiatric disturbances were identified in 28% of children referred to general paediatric clinics (Garralda & Bailey 1989). Two-thirds had an *emotional disturbance*.

In the NCDS at 7 years of age:

Maladjustment accounted for 27%
Deviant behaviour 71%
(Symptoms included withdrawal, depression, anxiety, restlessness, hostility, unforthcoming, 'writing people off '.)

In the IOW (Rutter 1970) at age 10–11 years:

Psychiatric problems – 7%,
Conduct disorders   – 4%
Emotional problems – $2\frac{1}{2}$

The disorders were associated with lower IQ, brain damage or associated physical disability whilst emotional problems were related to poor marital relationships, lack of warmth shown towards the children and a psychiatric history of one or other parent. In a study of schoolchildren by Shepherd et al (1971) an incidence of 4% *abnormal mood changes* and 10% *excessive crying* was found.

Boys have a higher deviance rate than girls (Hill 1986). In the NCDS, 16.9% of boys and 9.9% of girls were diagnosed as maladjusted whilst 41.9% of boys and 29.1% of girls showed an overall deviant behaviour; the IOW study showed a twofold excess of boys particularly in conduct disorders. The lower the social class of the heads of households the higher was the score of deviance of their children. Differences were found between city and country dwellers; for children in middle childhood living in cities 25% and 14% for children in the country (Graham 1986). In the city of Beijing, 9% of children aged 7–14 years had behaviour problems (Yu-feng 1989), boys showing a higher deviance, with antisocial behaviour predominating whilst girls were more likely to have neurotic behaviour. These behaviours are seen at home and school (Davie 1968, Davie et al 1971) and tend to persist (Baker et al 1983).

Adolescence

Adolescents have a prevalence rate of 20% for *significant psychological problems* (Graham 1986) and 1.4/1000 for *affective disorders* (Rutter et al 1976). 4% of 14–16-year-olds have a *depressive disorder*. In adolesence sex differences are not seen, girls having a similar prevalence of problems to boys.

DIAGNOSIS OF ABNORMAL PERSONALSOCIAL DEVELOPMENT

Personalsocial development is an important parameter in children's development and one which affects not only the whole child but often the whole family. Studying it is part of the everyday work of a DP and he has to decide when abnormalities are important or pathological enough to need further investigation.

Making the diagnosis

A wide knowlege and understanding of *normal* personalsocial development is the foundation for making a correct diagnosis of *abnormality*. Normal behaviour has a wide range, what is acceptable in one milieu is not in another, so the clinician has to take into account factors which may affect development. Taking a careful history may seem to be stating the obvious but less serious behavioural and emotional irregularities are often not volunteered by parents. Yudkin's (1961) account of 'teasing out' parental worries illustrates the importance of history taking. The history is best divided into *personal* and *social*.

Personal history

A history of eneuresis, encopresis, and sleep problems will be taken and the state of maturity of eating, sleeping and sphincter habits estimated. The child's temperament, behaviour and emotional reactions may be judged by direct questioning. Several clinical assessments have been devised to judge behavioural problems (Earls et al 1980, Jenkins et al 1980, Hodges & Tizard 1989). Observation during history taking may show overt abnormal behaviour in autism or lack of gaze in personal conversation in withdrawn girls (compared with aggressive girls) (Rutter & O'Brien 1980).

Questionnaires. There is a plethora of questionnaires to gauge temperament, behaviour and emotional problems in babies and children of all ages.

For young babies Brazelton (1973) scales have been devised but health visitors, using their own scheme, were equally as discerning (Sewell et al

1982). There are several for children of 4 months–7 years (Carey 1970, 1972, Fullard et al 1984, Devitt et al 1978).

For older children the Graham and Rutter parent interview (1968) proves useful. The Bristol social adjustment scales (Stott 1963) and the Vineland social maturity scales (1965) are quick and helpful although the latter are not reliable for young children and babies for whom a straightforward history is vastly superior.

Generally, the complicated lengthy questionnaires are more appropriate for use by psychologists but the DP needs to know what information they tap. Some questionnaires can be completed by other professionals, e.g. schoolteachers (Roper & Hinde 1979); nursery teachers (Scarlett 1980, Weir & Duveen 1981); parents (Achenbach et al 1987) and children (Achenbach et al 1987). Others tap social behaviour such as: reactions to strangers (Horner 1980); strange situations (Ainsworth et al 1978); listening skills (Friedlander et al 1974) and investigate special groups: autism (Krug et al 1980); disabled young adults (Trower et al 1978, Thomas & Bax et al 1988); aggression, delinquency and depression (Achenbach et al 1987); depression (Lang & Tisher 1980, Kazdin 1987). Gibbs et al (1987) question the issues of reliability and validity of many such questionnaires.

Estimating social development

Social behaviour might be seen in terms of behaviour with parents, siblings, the wider family, school and other milieux and these circumstances of the child will be enquired into. Although there are many checklists for estimating family stress (e.g. Metz et al 1976) direct questioning usually suffices. Behavioural problems are usually complained of by parents at home, school or both.

Analysing family relations

The Bene Anthony family relations test (1978)

For this test the child chooses, from amongst cardboard drawings, an imaginary family which corresponds to his own. These representational drawings are 'stood up' and have a small box behind them with a slit in it like a letter box. An extra drawing is of the back of a man called Mr Nobody. The child reads or has read to him, according to age, a card on which is written an attitude or emotion which is either incoming to or outgoing from other members of his family. The card is 'posted' into the box behind the drawing of the person to whom he considers it most applies. If no-one is identified the card is 'posted' into Mr Nobody. Later cards are added up and give an idea of the child's view of incoming and outgoing emotions. This test is helpful particularly in relationships between the child and his siblings. Jealousy or a feeling that parents discriminate between him and other children in the family have been the feelings most commonly discovered. Extra cards with symptoms relating to depression or sadness and the mother/father relationships can extend this test. A dramatic use of this test is described:

A $4\frac{1}{2}$-year-old girl was in hospital, the subject of child abuse. The abuser was not known, both parents denying any abuse. She was not speaking to the nursing staff. Alone in the playroom with the DP, she cooperated with developmental assessment and was of normal intelligence. She came from a large family. All siblings were discussed and appropriate cardboard pictures from the Family Relations test were chosen to represent them. She chose which drawing would represent mother but when it was suggested 'and now we must choose Daddy' her relaxed mood disappeared instantly. She did not want a daddy in her family she said. Eventually, after Mr Nobody had been introduced, she reluctantly agreed that he could represent 'Daddy' however he was to be quite separate from the rest of the family (Fig. 7.11). Several extra cards had been made out, such as: This is the one I am afraid of. This is the one who hits me. Mummy is frightened of this one. ALL negative incoming and outgoing feelings were posted into Mr Nobody. Eventually she became agitated and said she did not want to play any more.

At this time there was no evidence that father was the perpetrator, the child refusing to speak on the matter. Much later, when at a happy foster placement, the child told the truth but the results of the Family Relations test were the first evidence of who was the abuser. Eventually the father was convicted.

This highlights one of the advantages of a test in which children do not have to verbalize their feelings.

Abnormalities of personalsocial development: classification and associations

It is less easy nor desirable to divide children's behaviour into personal and social when considering a diagnosis. For example, the combination of emotional disturbances and abnormal family lifestyles spills into both personal and social parameters. Behavioural and emotional problems

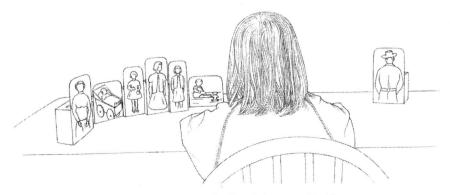

Fig. 7.11   Playing the family relations test. Daddy, as Mr Nobody, is separate from all the others.

ABSENT FROM SCHOOL

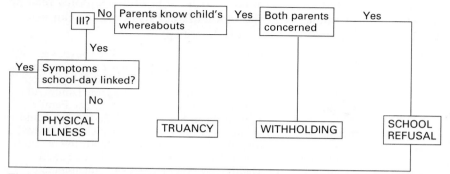

Fig. 7.12 Identification of 'absent from school' (from Hill P, Murray R, Thorley A (Eds) Essentials of Postgraduage Psychiatry. Grune & Stratton, London. Courtesy of Grune & Stratton).

differ with age so a knowledge of the phases of development is useful. The DP has to estimate severity of symptoms and recognize the rare psychoses when they present. For example, what distinguishes a child with a phobia of being abandoned by parents from what might be almost a normal developmental phase is the severity and duration of the phobia and how much it restricts the child's everyday life. 20% of school-children show some reluctance to go to school at times but less than 0.2% are likely to develop school refusal (Stewart 1980). Absence from

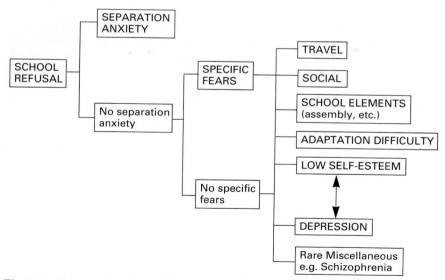

Fig. 7.13 School refusal (From Hill P, Murray R, Thorley A (Eds) Essentials of Postgraduage Psychiatry. Grune & Stratton, London. Courtesy of Grune & Stratton).

themselves. Psychiatrists may treat some conduct disorders by this method (Graham 1986). Another form of behaviour therapy is play therapy. Dolls, doll's houses and the creation of everyday situations are used in a psychoanalytical method which assumes that the child will 'play out' feelings and past events. Newsom et al (1979) describe a much more practical and developmental approach to play therapy.

Conditioning

Although a form of behaviour therapy it derives from classical conditioning. The bell and pad method of treating eneuresis is the only conditioning method in common practice but is of proven efficacy (Lansdown 1984, Hill 1986).

Teaching social skills

Training programmes in social skills may be for groups or individuals. Stroh et al (1986) describe the successful training of a group of disturbed and institutionalized children in a feeding programme which resulted in increased communication. Starza-Smith (1989) described a different skill-teaching scheme in a residential setting which was an adaptation of the Portage model (Shearer et al 1972), which is a home-based scheme which has proved successful for retarded and socially deprived children. It includes other developmental parameters as well as personalsocial. Isolated and rejected children, when given such training, were no more improved than those who received an 'attention' placebo or no-treatment (Tiffen & Spence 1986) but McCredie's study had very positive results. Polnay (1985) describes a service for problem families which is a combination of self-help, improving parenting skills and home economics which could be of considerable advantage to families.

Drugs

Drugs are not widely used in the treatment of personalsocial abnormalities, their use being mostly confined to the more severe psychiatric disorders. Occasionally a refractory case of enuresis may respond to a tricyclic antidepressant, usually Imipramine.

CONCLUSION

Personalsocial development is extremely important for the successful emergence of the growing child into society. Perhaps not enough attention is paid to helping children to do this successfully. This is a development much affected by environmental factors and the spreading of knowledge of factors which can affect this parameter to parents, teachers and all concerned with the care of children might have far-reaching effects. It could give children more personal happiness and increase their potential for a fulfilled and productive life.

REFERENCES

Achenbach T M, Verhulst F C, Baron G D, Althaus M 1987 A comparison of syndromes derived from the child behaviour checklist for American and Dutch boys aged 6–11 and 12–16. Journal of Child Psychology and Psychiatry and Allied Disciplines 28: 437–453

Ainsworth M D S 1967 Infancy in Uganda. Johns Hopkins University Press, Baltimore

Ainsworth M D S 1973 The development of the infant–mother attachment. In: Caldwell G B, Ricciuti H N (eds) Review of Child Development Research, vol 3. University of Chicago Press, Chicago

Ainsworth M D S, Blehar M, Waters E, Wall S 1978 Patterns of attachment. Erlbaum, New Jersey

Ali Z, Lowry M 1981 Early maternal–child contact: effects on later behaviour. Developmental Medicine and Child Neurology 23: 337–345

Arhens R 1954 Beitrag zur Entwicklung der Physiognomie und Mimikerkennes. Zeitschrift für Experimentelle und angewandte Psychologie 2: 412–454

Baker I, Hughes J, Street E 1983 Behaviour problems in children followed from 5–8.5–9 years of age and their relation to educational attainment. Child: Care, Health and Development 9: 339–348

Bandura A 1977 Social learning theory. Prentice–Hall, Englewood Cliffs, New Jersey

Bandura A, Walters R H 1959 Adolescent aggression through imitation of aggressive models. Journal of Abnormal Social Psychology 63: 575–582

Baruch G K, Barnett R C 1979 Fathers' participation in family work: a technical report. Working Paper 106. Wellesley College Center for Research on Women, Massachusetts

Batter B S, Davidson C V 1979 Wariness of strangers: reality or artifact? Journal of Child Psychology and Psychiatry and Allied Disciplines 20: 93–109

Bax M 1989 Eating is important. Editorial. Developmental Medicine and Child Neurology 31: 285–286

Bax M, Hart H 1976 Health needs of preschool children. Archives of Diseases in Childhood 51: 848

Bayley N 1932 A study of the crying of infants during mental and physical tests. Journal of Genetic Psychology 40: 306–329

Belsky J 1988 Infant day care and socioemotional development: the United States. Journal of Child Psychology and Psychiatry and Allied Disciplines 29: 397–406

Bene E, Anthony J 1978 Family Relations Test: an objective technique for exploring emotional attitudes in children. NFER–Nelson, Windsor

Bidder R T, Gray O P, Pates R M 1981 Brief intervention for behaviourally disturbed pre-school children. Child: Care, Health and Development 7: 21–30

Biller H B 1971 Father, child and sex role. Heath, Lexington, Massachusetts

Bohman M, Sigvardsson S 1979 Long-term effects of early institutional care: a prospective long-term longitudinal study. Journal of Child Psychology and Psychiatry and Allied Disciplines 20: 111–117

Boniface D, Graham P 1979 The three-year-old and his attachment to a special soft object. Journal of Child Psychology and Psychiatry and Allied Disciplines 20: 217–224

Bower T 1977 Artificial senses for handicapped children. In: Bruner J, Cole M, Lloyd B (eds) The perceptual world of the child. Fontana, London

Bowlby J 1958 The nature of the child's tie to his mother. International Journal of Psychoanalysis 39: 350–373

Bowlby J 1969 Attachment and loss. Vol 1. Attachment. Hogarth Press, London

Bowlby L J 1951 Maternal care and mental health. WHO, Geneva

Brazelton T B 1973 Neonatal behavioral assessment scale. J B Lippincott, Philadelphia

Brazelton T B 1979 Behavioural competence of the newborn infant. Seminars in Perinatalogy 3: 35–44

Breznitz Z, Friedman S L 1988 Toddlers' concentration: does maternal depression make a difference? Journal of Child Psychology and Psychiatry and Allied Disciplines 29: 267–279

British Medical Journal Leader. Helping mothers to love their babies. British Medical Journal 3.9.77: 595–596

Bronson W C 1975 Development in behavior with age mates during the second year of life. In: Lewis M, Rosenblum L A (eds) The origins of behavior: friendship and peer relations. Wiley, New York

Bryan E M 1983 The nature and nurture of twins. Baillière Tindall, London

Buss A H, Plomin R A 1975 Temperament theory of personality development. Wiley, New York

Campion J, Wohlfarth R 1989 Theory and research in practice: an opportunity group for young children with developmental difficulties. Child: Care, Health and Development 15: 343–361

Carey W B 1970 A simplified method for measuring infant temperament. Journal of Pediatrics 77: 188–194

Carey W B 1972 Measuring infant temperament. Journal of Pediatrics 81: 414

Clancy H, McBride G 1975 The isolation syndrome in childhood. Developmental Medicine and Child Neurology 17: 198–219

Coleman J, Wolkind S, Ashley L 1977 Symptoms of behaviour disturbance and adjustment to school. Journal of Child Psychology and Psychiatry and Allied Disciplines 18: 201–209

Coons S, Guilleminault C 1984 Development of consolidated sleep and wakeful periods in relation to the day/night cycle in infancy. Developmental Medicine and Child Neurology 26: 169–176

Cox A D, Puckering C, Pound A, Mills M 1987 The impact of maternal depression in young children. Journal of Child Psychology and Psychiatry and Allied Disciplines 28: 917–928

Crnic K A, Ragozin A S, Greenberg M T, Robinson N M, Basham R B 1983 Social interaction and developmental competence of preterm and full-term infants during the first year of life. Child Development 54(b): 1199–1210

Curtiss S 1977 Genie: a psycho-linguistic study of a modern-day 'wild child'. New York Academic Press, New York

Dansky J L 1980 Cognitive consequences of sociodramatic play and exploration training for economically disadvantaged preschoolers. Journal of Child Psychology and Psychiatry and Allied Disciplines 20: 47–58

Darwin C 1872 The expressions of the emotions in man and animals. (1965 edn., University of Chicago Press, Chicago)

Darwin C 1877 A biographical sketch of an infant. Mind 7: 285–294

Davie R 1968 The behaviour and adjustment of seven-year-olds. British Journal of Educational Psychology 38: 1–2

Davie R, Butler N, Goldstein H 1972 From birth to seven. Longman, London

Davie R, Butler N, Goldstein H 1972 From Birth to Seven: a Report of the National Child Development Study. Longman, London

Delaney E J 1965 Parental antecedents of social aggression in young children. Diss Abstr 26(3): 1763

Desmond M M, Wilson G S 1975 Neonatal abstinence syndrome: recognition and diagnosis. Addictive Diseases: An International Journal 2: 113–21

Devitt S C, Carey W B 1978 The measurement of temperament in 3–7-year-old children. Journal of Child Psychology and Psychiatry and Allied Disciplines 19: 245–253

Douglas J W B 1964 The home and the school. MacGibbon and Kee, London

Dunn J, Kendrick C, MacNamee R 1981 The reaction of first-born children to the birth of a sibling: mothers' report. Journal of Child Psychology and Psychiatry and Allied Disciplines 22: 1–18

Dunphy D C 1963 The social structure of urban adolescence peer groups. Sociometry 26: 236

Earls F, Richman N 1980 The prevalence of behavior problems in three-year-old children of West Indian-born parents. Journal of Child Psychology and Psychiatry and Allied Disciplines 21: 99–106

Efoghe G B 1987 In: Lamb M E (ed) The father's role: cross-cultural perspectives. Erlbaum, New Jersey

Efoghe G B 1987 Perception of parental punitiveness toward aggression as influenced by sex and socio-economic class in Efooma, Bendel State, Nigeria. Journal of Child Psychology and Psychiatry and Allied Disciplines 28: 847–854

Emde R N, Gaensbauer T J, Harmon R J 1976 Emotional expression in infancy. A biobehavioural study. International Universities Press, New York

Emde R N, Katz E L, Thorpe J K 1978 Emotional expression in infancy. 2. Early deviations in Down's syndrome. In: Lewis M, Rosenblum L A (eds) The development of affect. Plenum Press, New York

Epir S, Renda Y, Baser N 1984 Cognitive and behavioural characteristics of children with idiopathic epilepsy in a low-income area of Ankara, Turkey. Developmental Medicine and Child Neurology 26: 200–207

Erikson E H 1963 Childhood and society. Norton, New York

Eron L D, Lefkowitz M, Huesmann L A, Walder C O 1972 Does television violence cause aggression? American Psychology 27: 253–263

Foley H 1977 When do pre-term and light-for-dates babies smile? Developmental Medicine and Child Neurology 19: 5757–5760

Freedman D G 1965 Hereditary control of early social behaviour. In: Foss B M (ed) Determinants of infant behaviour, vol 3. Methuen, London

Freedman D G 1979 Ethnic differences in babies. Human Nature 2: 36–43

Freud S 1960 A general introduction to psychoanalysis. Washington Square Press, New York

Friedlander B Z, Wetstone H S, McPeek D L 1974 Systematic assessment of selective language listening deficit in emotionally disturbed pre-school children. Journal of Child Psychology and Psychiatry and Allied Disciplines 15: 1–12

Fullard W, McDevitt S C, Carey W B 1984 Assessing temperament in one- to three-year-old children. Journal of Paediatric Psychology 9: 205–217

Gallup G G Jr 1979 Self-recognition in chimpanzees and man: a developmental and comparative perspective. In: Lewis M, Rosenblum L A (eds) Genesis of behavior, vol 2. Child and its family. Plenum Press, New York

Garralda M E, Bailey D 1989 Psychiatric disorders in general paediatric referrals. Archives of Disease in Childhood 64: 1727–1733

Gehler W 1972 The development of social behaviour in pre-school and elementary grade children. Early Child Development and Care 1: 227–235

Gesell A 1954 The first five years of life. Methuen, London

Gesell A, Illg F, Ames A L, Rodell J 1946 Infant and child in the culture of today. Hamish Hamilton, London

Gewirtz J L 1965 The course of infant smiling in four child-rearing environments in Israel. In: Foss B M (ed) Determinants of infant behaviour, vol 3. Methuen, London

Ghodsian M, Zajicek E, Wolfind S 1985 Comparative study of social and family correlates of children's behaviour ratings. Child: Care, Health and Development 11: 209–228

Gibbs M V V, Reeves D, Cunningham C C 1987 The application of temperament questionnaires to a British sample: issues of reliability and validity. Journal of Child Psychology and Psychiatry and Allied Disciplines 28: 61–77

Glueck S, Glueck E 1962 Family environment and delinquency. Houghton Mifflin, Boston

Glueck S, Glueck G 1968 Delinquents and nondelinquents in perspective. Harvard University Press, Cambridge, Massachusetts

Goldstein A 1955 Aggression and hostility in the elementary school in low socio-economic areas. Understanding the Child 24: 20

Gomes-Pedro J, Almeida J B, da Costa C S, Barbosa A 1984 Influence of early mother–infant contact on dyadic behaviour during the first month of life. Developmental Medicine and Child Neurology 26: 657–666

Goodenough F L 1931 Anger in young children. Minnesota Press, Minneapolis

Goodyer I M, Wright C, Altham P M E 1988 Maternal adversity and recent stressful life events in anxious and depressed children. Journal of Child Psychology and Psychiatry and Allied Disciplines 29: 651–667

Gordon J, Smith E 1965 Children's aggression, parental attitudes and the effects of an affiliation-arousing story. Journal of Personality and Social Psychology 1: 654–659

Graham P 1974 Depression in pre-pubertal children. Developmental Medicine and Child Neurology 16: 340–349

Graham P 1984 Paediatric referral to a child psychiatrist. Archives of Disease in Childhood 59: 1103–1105

Graham P 1986 Child psychiatry: a developmental approach. Oxford Medical, Oxford

Graham P, George S 1973 Temperamental characteristics as predictors of behavioural disorders in children. American Journal of Orthopsychiatry 43: 328–339

Graham P, Rutter M 1968 The reliability and validity of psychiatric assessment of the child. ii. Interview with the parent. British Journal of Psychiatry 114: 581–592

Greene J G, Fox N, Lewis M 1983 The relationship between neonatal characteristics and three-month mother–infant interaction in high-risk infants. Child Development 54: 1286–1296

Griffin M, Hudson A 1978 Parents as therapists: the behavioural approach. PIT Press, Victoria

Hales D J, Lozoff B, Sosa R, Kennell J H 1977 Defining the limits of the maternal sensitive period. Developmental Medicine and Child Neurology 19: 454–461

Hart H, Bax M, Jenkins S 1984 Health and behaviour in preschool children. Child: Care, Health and Development 10: 1–16

Harter S 1982 The perceived competence scale for children. Child Development 53: 87–97

Hartup W W 1980 Peer relations and family relations: two social worlds. In: Rutter M (ed) Scientific foundations of developmental psychiatry. Heinemann Medical, London

Hebb D O 1946 On the nature of fear. Psychological Review 53: 259–276

Helms D B, Turner J S 1976 Exploring child behaviour. W B Saunders, Philadelphia

Helms D B, Turner J S 1976 Personality and social learning. In: Exploring child behavior. W B Saunders, Philadelphia

Herbert M 1987 Behavioural treatment of problems in children. In: Macfarlane J A (Ed) Progress in child health, vol 3. Churchill Livingstone, Edinburgh

Hewitt K, Hobday A, Crawford W 1989 What do health visitors gain from behavioural workshops? Child: Care, Health and Development 15: 265–275

Hill P 1986 Child psychiatry. In: Hill P, Murray R, Thorley A (eds) Essentials of postgraduate psychiatry. Grune & Stratton, London

Hill S D, Tomlin C 1981 Self-recognition in retarded children. Child Development 52: 145–150

Hoare P 1984 The development of psychiatric disorder among school children with epilepsy. Developmental Medicine and Child Neurology 26: 3–13

Hobson R P 1980 The question of egocentrism: the young child's competence in the co-ordination of perspectives. Journal of Child Psychiatry 21: 325–331

Hodges J, Tizard B 1989 IQ and behavioural adjustment of ex-institutional adolescents. Journal of Child Psychology and Psychiatry and Allied Disciplines 30.1: 53–75

Hodges K, McKnew D, Cytryn L, Stern L, Kline J 1982 The child assessment schedule (CAS) diagnostic interview: a report on reliability and validity. Journal of American Academy of Child Psychiatry 21: 468–473

Holmes S J, Robins L N 1987 The influence of childhood disciplinary experience on the development of alcoholism and depression. Journal of Child Psychology and Psychiatry and Allied Disciplines 28.3: 399–415

Horner T M 1980 Two methods of studying stranger reactivity. Journal of Child Psychology and Psychiatry and Allied Disciplines 21: 203–219

Hundleby J, Carpenter R, Ross R, Mercer G 1982 Adolescent drug use and other behaviours. Journal of Child Psychology and Psychiatry and Allied Disciplines 23.1: 61–68

Jarman 1985 Giving advice about welfare benefits in general practice. British Medical Journal 290: 522–524

Jarvelin M R 1989 Developmental history and neurological findings in enuretic children. Developmental Medicine and Child Neurology 31: 728–736

Jenkins S, Bax M, Hart H 1980 Behaviour problems in pre-school children. Journal of Child Psychology and Psychiatry and Allied Disciplines 21: 5–17

Jersild A T 1968 Child psychology, 6th edn. Prentice Hall, Englewood Cliffs, New Jersey

Jersild A, Markey F 1935 Conflicts between preschool children. Child Development Monographs No 21

Jones M B, Offord D R 1989 Reduction of antisocial behavior in poor children by nonschool skill-development. Journal of Child Psychology and Psychiatry and Allied Disciplines 30: 737–750

Kagan J 1971a Range and continuity in infancy. Wiley, New York

Kagan J 1971b Understanding children, behaviour, motives and thought. Harcourt Brace Jovanovich; New York

Kaila E 1932 The reactions of the infant to the human face. Ann.Univ.Abo. 17: 1–114

Kazdin A E 1987 Children's depression scale: validation with child psychiatric inpatients. Journal of Child Psychology and Psychiatry and Allied Disciplines 28: 29–41

Kennell J H 1974 Developmental Medicine and Child Neurology 16: 172

Kisker G 1972 The disorganised personality, 2nd edn. McGraw–Hill, Hightstown, New Jersey

Klaus M H, Jerauld R, Kregen N, McAlpine W, Steffa M, Kennell J H 1972 Maternal attachment: importance of the first postpartum days. New England Journal of Medicine 286: 460

Klaus M H, Kennell J H 1976 In: Hull D (ed) Recent advances in paediatrics, no 5. Churchill Livingstone, Edinburgh

Klaus M H, Plumb N, Zuehlke 1970 Human maternal behaviour at the first contact with her young. Pediatrics 46: 187

Krug D, Arick J, Almond P 1980 Behaviour checklist for identifying severely handicapped individuals with high levels of autistic behaviour. Journal of Child Psychology and Psychiatry and Allied Disciplines 21: 221–229

Lamb M E 1987 The emergent American father. In: Lamb M E (ed) The father's role. Cross-cultural perspectives. Erlbaum, New Jersey

Lambert L, Essen J, Head J 1977 Variations in behaviour ratings of children who have been in care. Journal of Child Psychology and Psychiatry and Allied Disciplines 18: 335–346

Lancaster S, Prior M, Adler R 1989 Child behavior ratings: the influence of maternal characteristics and child temperament. Journal of Child Psychology and Psychiatry and Allied Disciplines 30: 137–149

.Landry S H, Loveland K A 1988 Communication behaviours in autism and developmental language delay. Journal of Child Psychology and Psychiatry and Allied Disciplines 29: 621–634

Lane H 1977 The wild boy of Aveyron. Allen & Unwin, London

Lang M, Tisher M 1980 Children's depression scale. The Australian Council for Educational Research, Hawthorn

Lansdown B R 1984 Child development made simple. Heinemann Professional, Oxford

Lansdown B R 1984 Child development. Heinemann, London

Largo R H, Stutzle W 1977 Longitudinal study of bowel and bladder control by day and at night in the first 6 years of life.1. Developmental Medicine and Child Neurology 19: 598–606

Largo R H, Stutzle W 1977 Longitudinal study of bowel and bladder control by day and at night in the first 6 years of life. 2. Developmental Medicine and Child Neurology 19: 607–613

Levine M B 1975 Interparental violence and its effects on the children: a study of 50 families in general practice. Medicine, Science and the Law 15: 172–176

Lorenz K 1966 On aggression. Harcourt, New York

Lowenstein L F 1978 Who is the bully? The bullied and non-bullied child. Bulletin of the British Psychological Society 147–149: 316–318

Lynn R 1988 Educational achievement in Japan: lessons for the West. In: Anderson D (ed) Studies in social revaluation. Macmillan, London

Lytton H 1976 The socialization of 2-year-old boys: ecological findings. Journal of Child Psychology and Psychiatry and Allied Disciplines 17: 287–304

MacAuslan A 1975 Physical signs in association with depressive illness in childhood. Child: Care, Health and Development 1: 225–232

Maccoby C C 1980 Social development: psychological growth and the parent–child relationship. Harcourt Brace Jovanovich, New York

Maccoby E E, Jacklin C N 1974 The psychology of sex differences. Stanford University Press, Stanford, California

Maccoby E E, Jacklin C N 1980 Sex differences in aggression: a rejoinder and reprise. Child Development 51: 964–980

Maccoby E E, Masters J C 1970 Attachment and dependency. In: Mussen P H (ed) Carmichael's Manual of Child Psychology, 3rd edn. Wiley, New York

MacKeith R 1972 Is maturation delay a frequent factor in the origins of primary nocturnal enuresis? Developmental Medicine and Child Neurology 14: 217–223

MacKeith R 1973 The causes of nocturnal enuresis. In: Kolvin I, MacKeith R, Meadow S R (Eds) Bladder control and enuresis. Clinics in Developmental Medicine 48/49. Spastics International Medical Publishers/Heinemann Medical Books, London

MacLean C 1977 The wolf children. Penguin Books, Harmondsworth

Macredie T, Bradshaw J 1984 Teaching social skills: evaluation of an 'independence week'.

Child: Care, Health and Development 10: 181–188

Main M, Kaplan N, Cassidy J 1985 Security in infancy, childhood and adulthood: a move to the level of representation. In: Bretherton I, Waters E (eds) Monographs of the Society for Research in Child Development 50: 66–104

Martin B 1975 Parent-child relations. In: Horowitz F D (ed) Review of Child Development Research, vol 4. University of Chicago Press, Chicago

McDevitt S C, Carey W B 1978 The measurement of temperament in 3–7-year-old children. Journal of Child Psychology and Psychiatry and Allied Disciplines 19: 245–253

Meadow R 1984 Munchausen by proxy and brain damage. Developmental Medicine and Child Neurology 26: 669–676

Metz J R et al 1976 A pediatric screening examination for psychosocial problems. Pediatrics. 58: 595

Michelsson K, Rinne A, Paajanen S 1990 Crying, feeding and sleeping patterns in 1 to 12 month old infants. Child: Care, Health and Development 16: 99–111

Miller F, Court S, Walton W, Know E 1960 Growing up in Newcastle-upon-Tyne. Oxford University Press, Oxford

Minde K 1986 Bonding and attachment: its relevance for the present-day clinician. Developmental Medicine and Child Neurology 28: 803–805

Minde K, Minde R 1977 Behavioural screening of pre-school children: a new approach to mental health. In: Graham P (ed) Epidemiological approaches in child psychiatry. Academic Press, London

Morgan M 1982 Television and adolescents' sex-role stereotypes: a longitudinal study. Journal of Personality and Social Psychology 43: 947–955

Morris S E 1981 Communication/interaction development at mealtimes for the multiply handicapped child: implications for the use of augmentative communication systems. Speech XII: 216–232

Mussen P H, Jones M C 1957 Self-conceptions, motivations and interpersonal attitudes of late and early maturing boys. Child Development 28: 243–256

Neill S R St J 1982 Preschool design and child behaviour. Journal of Child Psychology and Psychiatry and Allied Disciplines 23.3: 309–318

Newsom J, Newsom E 1966 Rights and privileges of property and play. In: 4 years old in an urban community. Pelican Books, London

Newsom J, Newsom E, Head J, Mogford K 1979 Toys and playthings in development and remediation. Penguin Books, Harmondsworth

Nunn K 1986 Annotation. The episodic dyscontrol syndrome in childhood. Journal of Child Psychology and Psychiatry and Allied Disciplines 27: 439–446

Oates R K 1984 Personality development after physical abuse. Archives of Disease in Childhood 59: 147–150

Offord D R 1987 Prevention of behavioural and emotional disorders in children. Journal of Child Psychology and Psychiatry and Allied Disciplines 28: 9–19

Olweus D 1978 Aggression in the schools: bullies and whipping boys. Hemisphere, Washington

Oppel W, Harper P, Rider R 1968 Social, psychological and neurological factors associated with nocturnal enuresis. Pediatrics 42: 627–641

Ouelette E M, Rosett H L, Rosman N P, Weiner L 1977 Adverse effects of offspring of maternal alcohol abuse during pregnancy. New England Journal of Medicine 297: 528–530

Palti H, Zilber N, Kark S L 1982 A community-orientated early intervention programme integrated in a primary preventive child health service — evaluation of activities and effectiveness. Community Medicine 4: 302–314

Pearce J 1977 Depressive disorder in childhood. Child Psychiatry 18: 79–82

Pelligrine D S, Masten A S, Garmezy N, Ferrarese M J 1987 Correlates of social and academic competence in middle childhood. Journal of Child Psychology and Psychiatry and Allied Disciplines 5: 699–714

Peskin H 1973 Influence of the developmental schedule of puberty on learning and ego development. Journal of Youth and Adolescence 2: 273–290

Piaget J 1926 Studies in child logic, vol 1. Language and thought in the child. Kegan Paul, London

Piaget J 1932 The moral judgement of the child. Macmillan, New York

Piaget J 1953 The origins of intelligence. Routledge and Kegan Paul, London

Jersild A T 1969 Child psychology, 6th edn. Prentice–Hall, Englewoood Cliffs, New Jersey, p 317

Pichaud D 1979 The cost of a child. Poverty, pamphlet 43. Child Poverty Action Group, London

Plowden Report 1967 Children and their primary schools. HMSO, London

Pollak M 1979 Nine years old. MTP Press, Lancaster

Pollak M 1979 Today's three-year-olds in London. Heinemann, London

Pollak M 1984 Family practice and child development.In: Gray D J P, Gray J P (eds) The Medical Annual. The Year Book of General Practice. Wright, Bristol

Pollak M 1986 Father's involvement in child development. World Pediatrics and Child Care 3: 283–285

Pollak M 1988 Three years old around the world. Paper read to First International Meeting of Social Paediatrics, Munich, October 1988

Pollak M 1989 Social deprivation and language development: diagnosis and treatment. World Paediatrics and Child Care 4: 53–57

Pollak B 1989 Unpublished report

Polnay L 1985 Personal practice: a service for problem families. Archives of Disease in Childhood 60: 887–890

Pratt K C 1945 A study of the fears of rural children. Journal of Genetic Psychology 67: 179–194

Prechtl H F R, Beintema D J 1964 The neurological examination of the full term newborn infant. Clinics in Developmental Medicine 12: Spastics International Medical Publications, Heinemann Medical Books, London

Radin N 1982 Primary caregiving and role-sharing fathers. In: Lamb M E (Ed) Nontraditional families: parenting and child development. Erlbaum, New Jersey

Rheingold H L, Eckerman C D 1970 The infant separates himself from his mother. Science 168: 78–83

Richards M 1982 Do broken marriages affect children? Health Visitor 55: 152–153

Richards M P M 1984 Children and divorce. In: Macfarlane J A (ed) Progress in child health, vol 1. Churchill Livingstone, Edinburgh

Richardson S A 1976 Attitudes and behaviour toward the physically handicapped. In: Bergsma D, Pulver A E, Liss A R (eds) Developmental disabilities: psychological and social implications. New York

Richman N 1981 A community survey of characteristics of one- to two-year-olds with sleep disruptions. American Academy of Child Psychology 20: 281–291

Richman N 1985 Sleep disorders in young children. In: Macfarlane J A (ed) Progress in Child Health, Vol 2. Churchill Livingstone, Edinburgh

Richman N, Stevenson J E, Graham P 1982 Pre-school to school: a behavioural study. Academic Press, London

Richman N, Stevenson J, Graham P 1975 Prevalence of behaviour problems in three-year-old children: an epidemiological study in a London Borough. Journal of Child Psychology and Psychiatry and Allied Disciplines 16: 277–287

Rodholm M 1981 Effects of father–infant post-partum contact on their interaction: 3 months after birth. Early Human Development 5: 79–86

Rogers S J 1986 Assessment of infants and preschoolers with low-incidence handicaps. In: Lazarus P J, Strichart S S (eds) Psychoeducational evaluation of children and adolescents with low-incidence handicaps. Grune & Stratton, Orlando, Florida

Rogers S J, Puchalski C B 1984 Social characteristics of visually impaired infants' play. Topics in Early Childhood Special Education 3: 52–57

Roper E, Hinde R A 1979 A teacher's questionnaire for individual differences in social behaviour. Journal of Child Psychology and Psychiatry and Allied Disciplines 20: 287–298

Rosenthal M K 1967 Effects of a novel situation and of anxiety on two groups of dependency behaviours. British Journal of Psychology 58(3–4): 357–364

Russell A 1989 Guidelines in early integrative socio-educational interaction and play: from 18 months onwards. World Paediatrics and Child Care 4: 29–34

Rutter D R, O'Brien P 1980 Social interaction in withdrawn and aggressive maladjusted girls: a study of gaze. Journal of Child Psychology and Psychiatry and Allied Disciplines 21: 59–66

Rutter M 1972 Maternal deprivation reassessed. In: Foss B M (ed) Penguin science of behaviour. Penguin Books, Harmondsworth

Rutter M 1979 Maternal deprivation 1972–1978: new findings, new concepts, new approaches. Child Development 50: 283–305

Rutter M 1980 Emotional development. In: Rutter M (ed) Scientific foundations of developmental psychiatry. Heinemann, Oxford

Rutter M 1981 Stress, coping and development: some issues and some questions. Journal of Child Psychology and Psychiatry and Allied Disciplines 22: 323–356

Rutter M 1982 Prevention of children's psychosocial disorders: myth and substance. Pediatrics 70: 883–894

Rutter M L, Graham P, Yule W 1970 A neuropsychiatric study in childhood. Spastics International Medical Publishers/Heinemann Medical Books, London

Rutter M L, Quinton D, Yule B 1980 Family pathology and disorder in children. Wiley, London

Rutter M, Cox A, Tupling C, Berger M, Yule W 1975 Attainment and adjustment in two geographical areas. 1. Prevalence of psychiatric disorders. British Journal of Psychiatry 126: 493–509

Rutter M, Graham P, Chadwick O, Yule W 1976 Adolescent turmoil: fact or fiction? Journal of Child Psychology and Psychiatry and Allied Disciplines 17: 35–56

Rutter M, Shaffer D, Shepherd M 1975 A multiaxial classification of child psychiatric disorders. WHO, Geneva

Rutter M, Tizard J, Whitmore K 1970 Education, health and behaviour. Longman, London

Scarlett W G 1980 Social isolation from agemates among nursery school children. Journal of Child Psychology and Psychiatry and Allied Disciplines 21: 231–240

Scarr S, Salapatek P 1970 Patterns of fear development during infancy. Merrill–Palmer Quarterly 16: 53–90

Schaffer D R 1985 Developmental psychology: theory, research and applications. Brooks/Cole, Monterey, California

Schaffer D R 1985 The self and social development. In: Developmental psychology: theory, research and applications. Brooks/Cole, Monterey, California

Schaffer D R, Johnson R D 1980 Effects of occupational choice and sex-role preferences on the attractiveness of men and women. Journal of Personality 48: 505–519

Shaffer D, Gardner A, Hedge B 1984 Behavior and bladder disturbance of enuretic children: a rational classification of a common disorder. Developmental Medicine and Child Neurology 26: 781–792

Schaffer H R 1971 The growth of sociability. Penguin Modern Psychology Readings. Penguin, Harmondsworth

Schaffer H R, Emerson P E 1964 The development of social attachment in infancy. Monographs of Social Research in Child Development 29 (3, no 94)

Schowalter J E 1977 The modification of behavior modification. Pediatrics 59: 130–131

Sears R R, Maccoby E E, Levin H 1957 Patterns of child rearing. Row and Peterson, Evanston, Illinois

Seidel U P, Chadwick O F D, Rutter M 1975 Psychological disorders in crippled children: a comparative study of children with and without brain damage. Developmental Medicine and Child Neurology 17: 563–573

Sewell J, Tsitsikas H, Bax M 1982 Comparison of the Brazelton NBAS with Health Visitors' assessments of the nursing couple. Developmental Medicine and Child Neurology 24: 615–625

Shannon F T, Fergusson D M, Dimond M E 1984 Early hospital admissions and subsequent behaviour problems in 6-year-olds. Archives of Disease in Childhood 59: 815–819

Shearer M, Shearer D 1972 The Portage project: a model for early childhood education. Exceptional Children 39: 210–217

Sheldon W H 1940 The varieties of human physique. Harper & Row, New York

Shepherd M, Oppenheim A N, Mitchell S 1971 Childhood behaviour and mental health. University of London Press, London

Showers J 1984 Research on twins: implications for parenting. Child: Care, Health and Development 10: 391–404

Shwalb D W, Imaizumi N, Nakazawa J 1987 The modern Japanese father: roles and problems in a changing society. In: Lamb M E (ed) The father's role: cross-cultural perspectives. Erlbaum, New Jersey

Sigvardsson S, Bohman M, Cloninger C R 1987 Structure and stability of childhood personality: prediction of later social adjustment. Journal of Child Psychology and Psychiatry and Allied Disciplines 28: 929–946

Sostek A, Vietze P, Zaslow M, Kreiss L, van der Waals Rubenstein D 1981 Social context in caregiver–infant interaction: a film study of Fais and the United States. In: Field T, Sostek A, Vietze P, Liederman P H (eds) Culture and early interaction. Erlbaum, New Jersey

Starza-Smith A 1989 The Bereweeke skill-teaching system in a residential setting for children with severe and profound learning difficulties. Child: Care, Health and Development 15: 241–250

Steele B F, Pollak C B 1974 A psychiatric study of parents who abuse infants and small children. In: Helfer R E, Kempe C H (eds) The battered child. University of Chicago Press, Chicago

Stein A, Fairburn C G 1989 Children of mothers with bulimia nervosa. BMJ 299: 777–778

Stevenson J E, Hawcroft J, Lobascher M, Smith I, Wolff O H, Graham P J 1979 Behavioural deviance in children with early treated phenylketonuria. Archives of Disease in Childhood 54: 14–18

Stewart M A 1980 Personality and psychoneurotic disorders. In: Gabel S, Erickson M T (eds) Child development and developmental disabilities. Little, Brown and Co., Boston

Stott D H 1963 The Social Adjustment of Children. Manual to the British Social Adjustment Guide. University of London Press, London

Stroh K, Robinson T, Stroh G 1986 A therapeutic feeding programme. 1. Theory and practice of feeding. 2. Links with language and learning. Developmental Medicine and Child Neurology 28: 3–18

Sylva K 1989 Does early intervention work? Archives of Disease in Childhood 64: 1103–1104

Thomas A P, Bax M C O, Smyth D P L 1988 The social skill difficulties of young adults with physical disabilities. Child: Care, Health and Development 14: 255–264

Thomas A, Chess S 1977 Temperament and development. Brunner/Mazel, New York

Thomson G O B, Raab G M, Hepburn W S, Hunter R, Fulton M, Laxen D P H 1989 Blood lead levels and children's behaviour: results from the Edinburgh Lead Study. Journal of Child Psychology and Psychiatry and Allied Disciplines 30: 515–528

Tiffen K, Spence S H 1986 Responsiveness of isolated versus rejected children to social skills training. Journal of Child Psychology and Psychiatry and Allied Disciplines 3: 343–355

Tizard B, Rees J 1975 The effect of early institutional rearing on the behaviour problems and affectional relationships of four-year-old children. Journal of Child Psychology and Psychiatry and Allied Disciplines 16: 61–74

Townsend P 1981 Toward equality in health through social policy. International Journal of the Health Services 11: 63–75

Townsend P, Davidson N 1982 Inequalities in health (The Black Report). Penguin, Harmondsworth

Trower P, Bryant B, Argyle M 1978 Social skills and mental health. Methuen, London

Turnbull C M 1972 The mountain people. Simon & Schuster, New York

Van Baar A L, Fleury P, Ultee C A 1989 Behaviour in the first year after drug-dependent pregnancy. Archives of Disease in Childhood 64: 241–245

Van Taassel E 1984 Temperament characteristics of mildly developmentally delayed infants. Journal of Developmental and Behavioral Pediatrics 5: 11–14

Verhulst F C, Althaus M, Berden G F M G 1987 The child assessment schedule: parent–child agreement and validity measures. Journal of Child Psychology and Psychiatry and Allied Disciplines 28: 455–466

Vineland Social Maturity Scales 1965 American Guidance Services, Circle Pines, Minnesota

Walker E 1981 Emotion recognition in disturbed and normal children: a research note. Journal of Child Psychology and Psychiatry and Allied Disciplines 22: 263–268

Walzer S, Wolff P H, Bowen D et al 1978 A method for the longitudinal study of behavioural development in infants and children: the early development of XXY children. Journal of Child Psychology and Psychiatry and Allied Disciplines 19: 213–229

Watson J B, Rayner R 1920 Conditioned emotional reactions. Journal of Experimental Psychology 3: 1–14

Weber F, Woolridge M W, Baum J D 1986 An ultrasonographic study of the organisation of sucking and swallowing by newborn infants. Developmental Medicine and Child Neurology 28: 19–24

has become intellectual in quality, prediction is both possible and reliable. The measurement of adaptive development is mostly a clinical tool since modification of procedures is encouraged with an interest in *how* as well as *if* a child performs whilst modification of procedures is disallowed in intelligence tests.

Adaptive development, being a modification of nonverbal intelligence, needs inclusion in any developmental examination. For example, only the assessment of adaptive development in a child with retarded language enables the differential diagnosis between mental retardation and a language delay to be made. Tests of adaptive development differentiate between intelligent and mentally handicapped children because adaptive development (or nonverbal intelligence) is retarded in mentally retarded children but not in intelligent handicapped children. For example, it was in tests of visual sequential memory, visual association and visual closure (i.e. performance tests) that subnormal children performed least well compared with normal children (Marinosson 1974). Tests of adaptive development help to differentiate the socially-deprived-but-intelligent child from the mildly mentally retarded child (Pollak 1989). The next developmental stage of adaptive development is demonstrated and the socially-deprived-but-intelligent child learns immediately whilst the retarded child takes much longer or does not learn in one lesson.

Since tests of adaptive development tap similar skills to performance in IQ tests, another reason for measuring adaptive development in preschool children is that this parameter anticipates performance scores in IQ tests. What is the evidence for this statement?

- The case for the predictability of development tests was argued in Chapter 5 and adaptive development was the parameter with the highest predictability.
- Gesell tests of adaptive development correlated highly with the Wechsler Test (Dubowitz et al 1977).
- Adaptive and language tests (Gesell) at 2 years of age were both predictive of later achievements (Siegel 1981).
- Gesell adaptive tests at 3 years correlated highly with intelligence and reading comprehension at 9 years (Pollak 1979).
- Nonverbal tests are predictive of later mathematical or scientific ability (Hills 1957, Barakat 1951, Wrigley 1958).

THE DEVELOPMENT OF ADAPTIVE SKILLS

Brick building

There is hardly a child in the world who does not like handling bricks — even if only to throw them across the room or at the examiner! For this reason bricks are ideal for beginning developmental assessments. Bricks are not merely playthings, should be 2.5 cm in size and of the same colour. Skills with bricks go through definite developmental stages and, when carried out with precision and the response noted with an accurate clinical eye, definite deductions can be made about the child's developmental level.

Spontaneous play with bricks

Up to age *15 months*, bricks are taken up, transposed, dropped, handed to mother or swept off the tabletop. By *18 months* one brick can be put on top of another and until *3 years* the child likes to dismantle and repeat the action indefinitely. By *3 years* he makes a horizontal alignment of bricks. Interest in repetition is waning but he likes to make several towers. (Fig. 8.1). At *4 years* he makes complicated structures in the vertical and horizontal planes and these have different shapes the second time around. By *5 years* building is usually three-dimensional and includes several units but when finished he is eager for a different task. Even *after 5 years of age*, given many bricks, children are not above play-

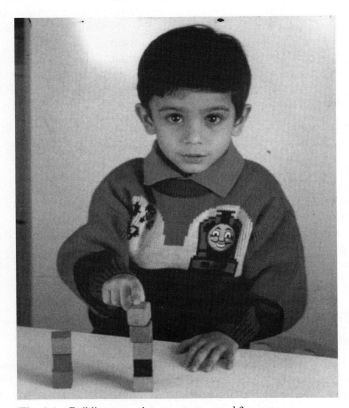

Fig. 8.1   Building more than one tower, aged 3 years.

ing with them and try intricate balancing acts or different constructional, almost architectural, tasks.

Offered bricks

The tabletop is clear, the examiner brings out bricks one by one, the child is given the correct number of bricks and no spare bricks are available.

By *4 months* a baby will reach out and take a proffered brick. Arm and hand movements go through developmental stages, thus from an initial arc movement of the whole arm there is gradually finer definition into separate hand and arm movements and eventual individual movement of each finger with maturation of grasp. Adaptive development looks for meaning in the action and the baby shows he understands that, if he reaches out to grasp an object, he can secure it. He knows that objects are separate from him and have position in space. *By 6 months* he can, in an instinctive reaction, take a brick in one hand and a second in the other. By *7–9 months of age* the *three-brick test* of adaptive development can be performed:

The baby, sitting on his mother's knee, has a brick held out to him in the midline. He takes and holds it tightly in one hand. The examiner offers another brick also in the midline. The baby takes this second brick in the other hand so one brick is firmly held in each hand. A third brick is offered. The baby will do one of the following:

- He will stare at the third brick with bewilderment (Fig. 8.2)
- He will look from hand to hand, each clutching its brick, look at the offered third brick and back to the two clutched bricks but does not attempt to take the third brick.
- He will drop one of his held bricks and take the third in this hand (Fig. 8.3). A variation is to drop one brick, transfer the second brick to the now free hand and take the third brick into the free hand.
- He retains a brick in each hand and attempts to take the offered brick in his mouth (Fig. 8.4).
- He will reach out and attempt to gather the three bricks in a cradle between his chest and hands
- He will try to take the brick in one or other hand and retain two bricks in one hand. If successful he is delighted with his achievement.
- He will transfer one brick to the other hand, either managing to retain or dropping the second and take the third one in the free hand. His sense of achievement shows clearly on his face.
- He may surprise by yet another individual response.

This is a wonderful example of adaptive development. The ability to reach out and take a brick is instinctive but there are the beginnings of intellectual processes in solving the problem of the third brick. His thought processes are seen by the way in which he 'adapts' the skills at his

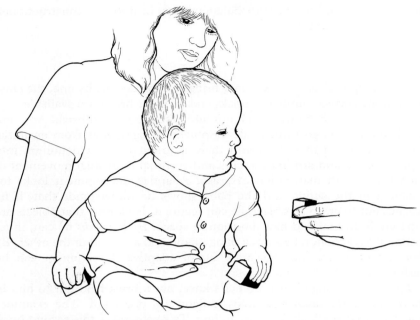

Fig. 8.2   Looking at the third brick.

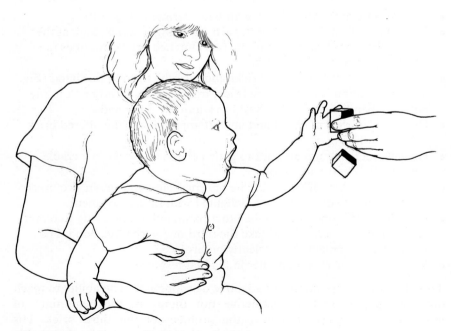

Fig. 8.3   Dropping second brick to take the third.

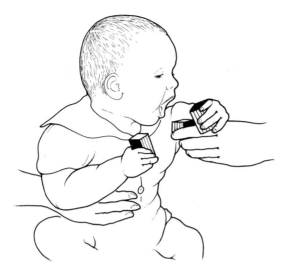

Fig. 8.4   Managing to hold all 3 bricks by mouthing.

command. Some severely environmentally deprived or mentally retarded babies deliberately look away as though pretending the situation does not exist, seeming unwilling to accept a problem either through fear of something unknown or a lack of zest for a testing situation. This might suggest that a zest for problem solving can be taught.

By *15 months* one brick is released upon another. This is an instinctive reaction. The increase in tower size is dependent upon motor agility and balance. Building a tower of three is present in 100% of normal *2-year-olds*, and a four-brick tower in 100% of normal *3-year-olds* (Gesell 1946). Most children are capable of much higher towers. In 392 children of different ethnic groups around the world 59% of 3-year-olds were able to build a tower of nine bricks (Fig. 8.5) and 81% built one of eight bricks (Pollak 1988). By $2\frac{1}{2}$ *years* he may make a horizontal line of bricks if given a demonstration and does so spontaneously by *3 years*. The skill of placing bricks horizontally is probably instinctive although mentally retarded children often reveal delay by continuing to put one brick upon another after the age at which this should cease.

Later brick building skills:

A train (Fig. 8.6) is made, preferably out of reach, in front of the child with an ongoing explanation. The train is moved along with a quiet 'choo-choo' sound. A *3-year-old*, given the correct number of bricks, should be able to make a train and push it along thereby showing that he can symbolize and (if he repeats the sound) that he heard. This test is more complicated than previous ones, involving combination of the vertical and horizontal which the child had so far learnt only as separate entities and he needs to conceptualize the shape as a moveable 'train'. This develop-

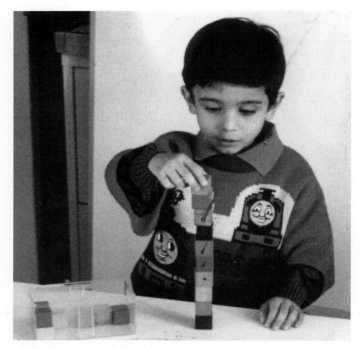

Fig. 8.5   Tower of 10 bricks, aged 3 years.

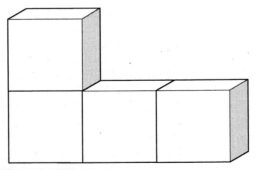

Fig. 8.6   Brick train.

mental level is paralleled exactly in the level of symbolic play possible at this age. It is at this stage that the divide between normal, average and mentally retarded children begins to show. A severely retarded child will be either unable to construct a horizontal line or still be making towers of one brick upon another and may be destructive and throw the bricks.

House (Fig. 8.7). The space between the two bricks and the placing of the brick over the 'hole' is pointed out. At $3\frac{1}{2}$ *years*, given the correct number of bricks, he copies this shape. An adaptation is .. 'This is a button in response to an order. Children are unable to use the train audiometer (see Ch. 11) or the Pollak tapper (Pollak & Tuchler 1982) before $5\frac{1}{2}$ *years* for the same reason. Highly gifted young children impress by their power of intense concentration. Rosvold et al (1956) have designed a useful test — the Continuous Performance Test — to discriminate between brain-damaged and normal children (and adults) which is based on the need for continuous attention.

Visuospatial perception

The relationship of visuospatial perception to adaptive development is not clear. One can see without perceiving and it is the *interpretation* of light waves falling upon the retina which is a cerebral function. Visual preference (and thus choosing) begins early in life but memory rather later but, when depth and space are perceived and memory is present, object permanence is recognized. Perception is aided by the natural tendency to group or class objects but is dependent upon attentiveness to the stimulus (Beadle 1970). That perception is improved by maturity is shown by the increasing ability with age of children to notice details embedded in a picture. Children are over 6 years before they can copy the geometric shape of Figure 8.14 (Gesell et al 1946) However, if the pattern is analysed for them, i.e showing how the rectangle is drawn, the cross inside and the corners joined with diagonal lines, children of 5 years are able to draw it although they are not mature enough to see this detail for themselves. Thus, perception is involved in adaptive development and many believe that visuomotor development is important for learning to read and spell. Abnormalities or delay in input of sensory information lead to poor motor development (Hogg 1982) and may be associated with learning difficulties. This was not the case in two children with Moebius Syndrome, who had poor motor integration and visual perception, but both had reading and arithmetic levels appropriate for their overall high IQs (Stebbins et al 1975, Kalverboer et al 1970).

Tests of adaptive development

The preschool child

Adaptive tests for the preschool child include: brick play; formboards and other puzzles; drawing; tests of memory, counting and attention span. These are usually sufficient to measure adaptive development in different areas and the DP will find them adequate. Other tests which may be helpful in certain circumstances include the following:

The Bus Puzzle Test (Egan & Brown 1984) has been standardized for an age range of 18 months to $4\frac{1}{2}$ years and has percentile charts of achievement in shape recognition and orientation of pieces. 90% of children aged *39 months* could select the recess for all 9 pieces. Although not a comprehensive test of adaptive development, the Bus Puzzle test has the advantage of measuring verbal and nonverbal ability in the same test and shows when children have wide differences between their verbal and performance skills.

The Trankell test of laterality (Trankell 1950) includes 20 items to measure an 'impulse scale'. Unfortunately, it is only scored for ages 7 to $10\frac{1}{2}$ years but is useful for this age range.

The Snijders-Oomen nonverbal intelligence test (1976), originally devised for deaf children, can be used as a test of nonverbal intelligence in normal children with a range of $2\frac{1}{2}$–7 year olds. For $2\frac{1}{2}$–7-year-olds there are: sorting, copying patterns, jigsaw-like shapes to place together, drawing simple shapes and finding a hidden object (memory) tests. Correlation is high with other IQ tests such as the Raven's progressive matrices and WISC. Although an excellent test it needs two hours to complete, which makes it unsuitable for the busy DP and small children prefer Gesell tests of adaptive development because there is continual change of material.

School age children

Raven's Progressive Matrices (Raven 1956). These tests are excellent for use by the DP being quick and enjoyed by children. Reasoning ability is measured by use of forms, patterns and shapes. The test consists of a patterned rectangle in which there is a hole. Underneath are six shapes, all of which fit into the hole but only one of which completes the pattern. The child has to choose which one it is. Initially, the choice is purely one of design but becomes increasingly complex and a point is reached at which choice is made by understanding the principle (i.e. intellectualizing). This taps a more complex problem-solving skill. The matrices can be used to diagnose intelligent children with specific learning difficulties (see Ch. 10). Intelligent children with visuospatial difficulties make many mistakes at the beginning of the series but often answer correctly those tests which can be intellectualized. This clinical use of the test greatly extends its range. There are four versions for different ages:

- A **coloured** set for children and the mentally handicapped (aged 6–85 yrs) which takes 7–10 minutes to administer. Raw scores can be converted to a percentile ranking.
- A **standard** set for $6\frac{1}{2}$ years to 65 years.
- An **advanced** type for 11 years upwards including adults.
- A **board** type (Raven 1956) for $3\frac{1}{2}$– 4-year-olds. These have been described as suitable for autistic children (Clark & Rutter 1979) and mentally retarded children. Each 'page' of patterns is made of cardboard and the individual shapes (also cardboard) fit into the hole of the large shape.

discharges fare least well (Stores et al 1976). Anticonvulsant drugs at toxic levels can cause a fall in intelligence especially nonverbal skills (Corbett et al 1985, Addy 1987). If the seizures are controlled there is usually little further deterioration 5 years later (Rodin et al 1986).

Idiopathic infantile hypercalcaemia is a rare disease (1 in 50 000 live births) associated with mental handicap but several papers have noted an inferiority of visuospatial and motor abilities compared with verbal skills in affected children. They have a high rate of behavioural disturbances (Udwin et al 1987, Martin et al 1984).

Craniopharyngioma. An intellectual deficit may follow the surgical removal of this tumour and a specific deficit in performance compared with verbal intelligence has been described (Clopper et al 1977, Galatzer et al 1981).

Chronic solvent abuse. Zur & Yule (1990) report a study of males with a history of chronic abuse of toluene and compare them with 12 delinquent boys. The solvent users tended to have lower overall intelligence scores but were particularly poor on symbol digit coding and were less accurate and slower on other tests of performance; these results do seem to suggest that chronic solvent abusers suffer a cognitive deficit which particularly affects nonverbal performance.

Albinism. There was a large verbal/performance discrepancy in favour of verbal skills in albino children whose intelligence quotients were in the normal range and when compared with a group of equally visually impaired children who were not albino. It is thought that the unusual visual pathways which albino children possess could be the explanation (Cole et al 1987).

Lead poisoning has been associated with visuospatial problems. Most studies show the intelligence quotient sustained but school performance falls off due to lack of attention and visuospatial problems (Chisholm & Barltrop 1979). There are problems in measuring chronic exposure to lead and not all authorities are agreed on these findings (Archives of Disease in Childhood 1980).

Turner syndrome. There is no agreement on the deficit of cognition in this syndrome. Originally it was thought that patients were globally retarded but several workers (Cohen 1957, Shaffer 1962, Silbert et al 1977) have demonstrated a large difference between verbal and performance scores on WISC and other tests in favour of verbal scores, the patients having poor visual memories. Waber (1979) confirmed poor visual memory and motor coordination although he failed to find clear evidence of a spatial ability deficit. It was thought that the loss of the X chromosome affected the visuospatial skills in Turner's syndrome but Ebbin et al (1980) have demonstrated poor skills in draw-a-man, Bender-Gestalt and visuo-motor tasks in mosaicism including the Y chromosome.

Mixed gonadal dysgenesis (45X/46,XY), being similar to Turner syndrome, is also associated with poor adaptive development.

Fragile X syndrome. Visualmotor integration is the problem most consistently present in *boys* with this syndrome (Dykens et al 1987).

Williams syndrome has been associated with special difficulties in visual reception, closure and memory — i.e. visuospatial tasks — compared with children of nonspecific developmental disabilites but matched for age, sex and global IQ (Crisco et al 1988).

CONCLUSION

Nonverbal or adaptive development has been shown by Gesell, Piaget and many intelligence tests to have many similar features. There is no doubt that intellect is concerned not only with language but also nonverbal or adaptive skills. Concept of numbers, mathematics and science are essentially nonverbal, adaptive skills. Although it is not possible to undertake one single test to measure adaptive development, it is essential to attempt assessment. Many children — and adults — do not have verbal and nonverbal skills in equal measure and it is important to have knowledge of marked differences. It appears that the environment plays a very much higher part in the acquisition of language than in adaptive skills. Cavemen drew and depicted their world long before they wrote books of their spoken language. The inadequacy of the language of children reared in silent worlds has already been mentioned yet Itard was able to teach Victor 'look-and-say' reading and to understand numerals (Lane 1977).

REFERENCES

Addy D P 1987 Cognitive function in children with epilepsy. Developmental Medicine and Child Neurology 29: 394–404

Archives of Disease in Childhood 1980 (Editorial) Children and lead: some remaining doubts. 55: 497–499

Barakat M K 1951 A factorial study of mathematical abilities. British Journal of Educational Psychology 4: 137–156

Beadle M 1970 A child's mind. How children learn during the critical years from birth to age five years. Methuen, London

Bee H 1981 The developing child. Harper International, New York

Binet A, Simon T 1916 The development of intelligence in children. Williams & Wilkins, Baltimore

Birch H G, Belmont L 1965 Auditory-visual integration in brain-damaged and normal children. Developmental Medicine and Child Neurology 7: 135

Bourgeois B F D, Prensky A L, Palkes H S, Talent B K, Busch S G 1983 Intelligence in epilepsy: a prospective study in children. Annals of Neurology 14: 438–444

Brunner R L, Berch D B, Berry H 1987 Phenylketonuria and complex spatial visualization: an analysis of information processing. Developmental Medicine and Child Neurology 29: 460–468

Chisholm J J, Barltrop D 1979 Recognition and management of children with increased lead absorption. Archives of Disease in Childhood 54: 249–262

9. Language development

Language — 'inner' linguistic skill and verbal intercourse — is one of the great attributes which distinguishes man from animals, many of whom have communication skills but no language.

How language is acquired is the subject of debate. One influence has been Chomsky (1957, 1959, 1969) who argues that infants have an inherent ability to acquire language. He bases his thesis on the following facts:

1. Language is acquired early
2. Language occurs in all cultures
3. People with almost any level of intelligence can speak
4. Without an inherent ability babies would never be able to distinguish language from the many sounds in the environment.

Moerk's theory (1977), on the other hand, has a more Piagetian basis, stating that a cognitive structure is inherent and can be applied to several media including language. Language is for man, not man for language.

Adults adopt differing attitudes towards babies and grownups. Eye contact is established early and lasts longer (Korner 1974), facial expression is exaggerated and pitch raised, 'babytalk' which is shorter, slower and repeated more often than adult talk, is adopted but there is the tacit acceptance that the baby is a human being (Costello 1977). All these attitudes help the baby to know that he is the centre of attention and help him to respond. Thus the social aspect and neuro-cognitive components of language acquisition combine. Infants possess auditory perception, voice and crude communication skills (Schlesinger & Meadow 1972) and the organization of linguistic skills is both cognitive and social.

There is ample evidence that language is a *learned* skill (Clark & Clark 1976, Davis 1947, Kolucjova 1972, Suzman 1958). Several centuries BC Psamethicus (Herodotus) reared two children apart from adults to see whether they would develop speech. They did not. The late Truffaut's enchanting film '*L'enfant sauvage*' is a visual evocation of a boy who was wild and nonverbal. It is based on the true story of the Wild Boy of Aveyron (Lane 1977) who never learned to communicate properly despite the inspired help he received from Jean-Marc Itard, a physician. If language is a *learned* skill acquisition will depend heavily on the environment. To have someone — especially a loved one — who both talks and listens, is benefit indeed for any growing child. Prelinguistic skills, the first aspects of communication, require the cooperation of another party. The interlocking of gaze, the smiling and crying which lead to the exchange of information are the first means of communication. The behaviour of adults in these situations has been described as a 'language teaching device' (Arkell 1983). Alternatively, to be acquainted with an essentially restrictive, repetitive and non-explanatory vocabulary, voiced by a variety of busy, uninvolved persons, or to be deprived opportunities for inter-communication, are known causes of linguistic disadvantage. Adults are the best teachers of language and children learn to talk and communicate from grown-ups rather than other children and nowhere is this more marked than in the prelanguage stages. A greater volume of language is heard by a child at home than at nursery school (Tizard et al 1976). The language of severely speech-delayed twins improved when they were separated and given parallel intensive language training (Douglas & Sutton 1978). The prescription of mixing with other children, whilst desirable for other reasons, is not correct treatment for language delay.

DEVELOPMENT OF LANGUAGE

The study of language development has been helped by studies which have demonstrated that language goes through developmental stages according to regular rules. Babies begin communicating soon after birth and the cries of pain and hunger are different even by a few days of life (Wolff 1969, Wasz-Hockert et al 1968). Frequency of crying differs between babies. Some cry little but whether these babies will develop language later than average or whether hyperactive children cry more is not known. Bax (1975) suggests a study of the cry might be used as: identification of abnormal babies, monitoring sick infants especially after anoxia, prognosis for recovery from brain damage and a quick diagnosis of some abnormalities. Excessive crying may be associated with disturbed mother–child relationships and perhaps provoke battering (Bernal 1972, Ounsted et al 1974, Bell & Ainsworth 1972). In order to develop language, babies need to hear and focus attention on human sounds (i.e. listen), interpret meanings from sounds and to produce signals and sounds of ever increasing sophistication. Feeding, nappy changing and bathing become times for communication.

Sequences of language development

3–5 months
— Attends to sounds especially parents' voices
— Babbles (essentially vowel sounds)
— Different cries and squeals for different emotions

4–7 months
— Listens to and localizes sounds
— Begins to understand the emotional overtones of language of familiar caregivers
— Begins to signal (e.g. putting arms up or excitement at the sight of food)
— Imitation of sounds, two-syllable sounds and a few consonants

8–10 months
— Listens preferentially to a sung nursery rhyme rather than a repeated tone (Glenn et al 1981)
— prefers a familiar rhyme to the same rhyme and intonation and stress patterns but with words reversed (Glenn & Cunningham 1982)

11–16 months
— Reacts to nearby meaningful sounds, especially from parents
— Responds appropriately to emotional overtones
— First spontaneous words used with meaning
— Tuneful jargon and 'trying out' of sounds
— Some echolalia

21–24 months
— Understands many words
— Carries out simple commands
— Vocabulary of 50 words
— Begins putting words together
— Echoes — immediate or delayed type
— Articulation is often indistinct
— Can symbolize lifesize objects and toys
— Song patterns become coherent and plays with musical toys

3 years
— Understand 60–80% of adult speech
— Understands semantic differences
— Vocabulary of 200 words
— Makes sentences of 3–4 words
— Symbolizes miniatures
— Undertakes two-part requests (Put dolly on chair)
— Asks questions
— Sings melodies and repeats rhymes
— May have absolute pitch (Ostwald 1973)

4–5 years
— Understands adult conversation except if content outside experience
— Has a wide vocabluary
— Uses correct grammar
— Some immatures of expression, especially 's' 'sh' 'th' and 'w'

— Plays and talks make-believe
— Questions everything

6–7 years
— Language is mature at home and outside and only higher intellectual content not understood
— Understands rules of games and turn-taking
— Language is intelligible and grammatically correct
— Retells happenings, stories and knowledge and has vivid imagination
— Beginning to read aloud.

FACTORS WHICH AFFECT LANGUAGE DEVELOPMENT

Position in family

The eldest child is the one most likely to have advanced language and the youngest child in a large family to have delayed language.

Twins

The development of language in twins is likely to be slower than singletons (Puckering & Rutter 1987, Douglas et al 1978, Illingworth 1987) due, in part, to twins interacting more with each other than with their parents — another example that language is predominantly learnt from adults.

Sex

Why boys are later in developing all aspects of language development, expressive language in particular, is not known but this is so (Howling & Rutter 1987).

Parents

To have a mother, parents or major single caregiver who gives time; who interacts verbally; who stimulates replies; who is prepared to listen; to tell stories or read books to the child are all factors known to enhance language development (Cazdan 1974, Hewison & Tizard 1980, Feitelson 1972, Dunn et al 1977). Delayed language development is associated with a young mother who smokes (Butler & Golding 1986); with depressed mothers (Cox et al 1987, Cohn et al 1986). Language development in hearing children with deaf mothers has been studied with inconclusive results. Some children have language problems whilst others do not. Some (e.g. Schill 1979) have reported delayed language in early childhood but later language was normal. Others (e.g. Schiff-Myers 1982) have not found the children's language to be affected at all.

Bishop (1979) has made out a good case for these subdivisions not being specific entities but rather lying upon a continuum with mild expressive delay at one end and severe developmental disorder at the most affected end. Bishop (1979) based her theory on research in which she demonstrated that children who appeared to have only an expressive problem — if given sophisticated investigative material which later included her own TROG (1983) — also have a problem of comprehension. The children studied were of school age and attending a special school for language disordered children and had they been tested at an earlier age no doubt their comprehension would have been found as affected as their expressive language. This does not invalidate Bishop's theory but rather points to the complicated nature of language disorders and to the fact that these disorders, like the children suffering them, develop and change with time.

Developmental language problems are of increasing severity:

a. Mild expressive delay

- The child understands to an age appropriate level all that is said to him
- Symbolic language is good
- Articulation is immature
- Vocabulary is poor
- Phonation may or may not be affected.

This is the most common language delay, much more common in boys and has a good prognosis.

b. Moderate expressive delay

- Vocabulary is poor
- Sentences are short and ungrammatical
- The child is incomprehensible to strangers although his mother may understand half of what he says
- Phonation is poor
- Symbolic language is good
- There are problems of comprehension in preschool years but comprehension is in advance of expression
- Boys are more affected than girls.

These are the children who, unless given specialist help, arrive at school unable to benefit to full potential and who have been so graphically described in the National Child Development Study.

c. Delay in comprehension

- Comprehension of language is delayed to a varying degree
- Language is that of a younger child

- Language is NOT abnormal
- Symbolic language is usually immature for chronological age (Fig. 9.1 shows a language delayed 4-year-old with immature symbolic language who is only able to symbolize a lifesize but not a miniature telephone)
- Boys are more affected than girls.

These children invariably have a delay in expressive language of less severity than the delay in comprehension. They need expert help and often have associated learning and behaviour problems at school age.

Language disorder

- Language is severely delayed and deviant
- History of abnormal preverbal development seldom obtained
- Comprehension affected more than expression
- Vocabulary extremely limited
- Utter many words often inappropriately

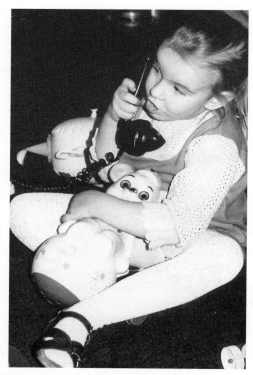

Fig. 9.1   Poor symbolic language; 4-year-old has to use adult telephone.

- Phonation is usually good
- Symbolic language totally absent.
- Deviance shown as frequent echolalia, usually of the immediate and rarely of delayed type (Dyer & Hadden 1981) the latter tending to the egocentric and inappropriate (Cantwell et al 1978)
- Phrases used are often associative (e.g. a little girl, being shown the daisy from the Reynell test (1969) began to sing, tonelessly 'Ring-a-ring of roses'; jingles from television advertisements may be correctly produced and their association definable)
- Often obsessional traits and repetitive behaviour. (Fig. 9.2)

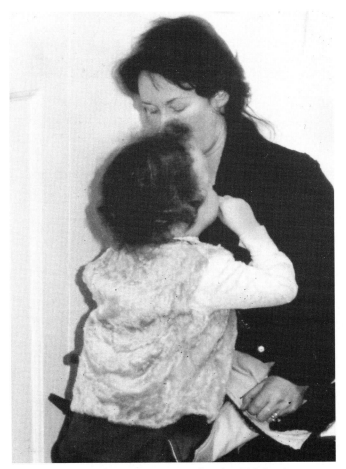

Fig. 9.2   Obsessional traits in language disorder. This boy is obsessional about furry material. His mother has made him a waistcoat of a special fur material and he is licking the fur collar of her coat.

- Usually eye contact with adults but not with other children
- Sex ratio is equal
- Adaptive skills are normal but deteriorate
- Gender identity is deficient (Abelson 1981).

When these features are accompanied by abnormal behavioural and emotional reactions and one accepts Bishop's concept of a continuum, it is easy to think that autism might be at the extreme end of such language continuum. However, Cantwell et al (1978) showed the language of 10-year-old autistic children to be different to that of severe 'developmental dysphasia'. Medical and neurological examinations, EEGs, MRI and CAT scans fail to reveal any abnormalities in these children, nor is there evidence of biochemical changes (Ritvo 1977). There have been rare reports of children with language disorder without fits whose EEGs showed bilateral or focal spike waves (Maccario et al 1982), but these are the exceptions. Some children with language disorders have mild delays in motor development (Bishop & Edmundson 1987) and problems of manipulation, locomotor function and musculature of speech apparatus (Sonksen 1977).

This is a severe condition with a poor prognosis requiring specialized treatment. Expressive language tends to improve with age but there is a paucity of underlying complicated linguistic cognitive concepts.

Acquired developmental language conditions of known aetiology

Temporary aphasia

This is an unusual phenomenon in idiopathic epilepsy which is transient but may recur with further fits.

Acquired aphasia (Wernicke type)

This aphasia usually follows an acute, unilateral (usually left) hemispheric lesion. The aetiology is more commonly post-traumatic but may be infective, vascular or neoplastic (Van Hout et al 1985). Young children have poor motor production, mutism and make a more rapid and better recovery than adults (Guttman 1942, Alajouanine & Lhermitte 1965).

Landau-Kleffner Syndrome

This is an acquired dysphasia usually associated with fits. An extremely rare condition — Landau & Kleffner (1957) described six cases whilst Cooper & Ferry (1978) and Bishop (1985) had difficulty when reviewing the world literature in finding 45 cases — but later Gordon (1990) reported 119 cases. It has gained attention mostly because of abnormal EEG findings which are so noticeably lacking in the developmental dysphasias.

Early language development is normal but later there is a profound loss of comprehension and a less marked loss of expressive language. Onset of fits is usually concurrent with or shortly after the onset of the condition. Motor, nonverbal and neurological examination are normal but EEGs show bilateral paroxysmal discharges with spike wave activities. Bishop (1982) has shown that language is deviant. Cromer (1978) described the condition as auditory agnosia, the language disorder resembling that of the profoundly deaf child although children are not cortically deaf. There is no agreement as to whether sign and written language are affected (Rapin et al 1977, Bishop 1982) which is unfortunate because if not some indication for treatment would be possible. Treatment with anticonvulsants is not usually beneficial. Prognosis is variable.

Acquired dysarthria

Most descriptions of dysarthria concern adults (Darley et al 1969) and those affecting children are usually congenital conditions such as cerebral palsy; however Bak et al (1983) describe an acquired type which followed a brainstem infarct in a 6-year-old boy. A breathy, nasal voice was noted together with distorted vowels and consonants.

Developmental speech defects of unknown aetiology

Stuttering

Stuttering is a dysrhythmia of speech due to incoordination of articulatory and respiratory function. Explanations are many, particularly in relation to bilateral speech representation (Jones 1966) but none convincing. The aetiology is largely unknown. Some 3–5-year-olds go through a normal developmental stage of stuttering and some have argued that this is exaggerated or prolonged in some children (Johnson 1959, Metraux 1950, Cave 1977). Stuttering occurs predominantly in boys (4:1), a positive family history is common (Andrews & Harris 1964) as is an association with late language development. An incidence of 1% in the school population and 9% in schools for the educationally subnormal was found in Newcastle. When stuttering causes distress and anxiety the condition needs treatment. Stages in stuttering have been described (Bloodstein 1960a) and are helpful in deciding when and how to treat.

ABNORMAL SPEECH AND LANGUAGE OF KNOWN AETIOLOGY

Sensory defects are of four main types: associated with deafness; blindness or partial sightedness; blindness with deafness; extreme environmental deprivation.

Language and deafness

Congenital deafness or deafness acquired in very early life has a different language development pattern to normal. Deafness of central origin has no babble but in other forms of deafness even profoundly deaf babies babble and continue to do so longer than is normal. When words fail to develop the babble dwindles — an interesting observation on the importance and possible role of preverbal communication in language development. Even more interesting is the observation (Freeman & Blockberger 1987) that the babbling, gesturing and understanding of deaf babies whose mothers are also deaf is better than that of deaf babies with hearing mothers (90% of cases) and is particularly so if the deaf mother is good at signing. Hearing parents depend on normal visual gesturing which is relatively undeveloped in these babies. Children who cannot hear are likely to have unintelligible speech but whether their language is delayed or deviant is a matter of debate. The language of mildly deaf children is surprisingly adequate for everyday use but most have later reading and spelling problems at school (Martin & Moore 1979, Critchley 1967). Profoundly deaf (loss >60dB) children are late in acquiring words and sentences, the latter are shorter and simpler than their hearing peers (Quinn & Macauslan 1986). They have articulatory and voice control problems and make semantic and syntactical errors. Resultant poor listening skills lead to inadequate comprehension and poor auditory memory. When deaf children are intelligent they are very good at gesturing and their symbolic language and play are good although some (e.g. Furth 1966, Furth & Youniss 1976, Conrad 1979) have noted later deficient symbolic reasoning.

A distinction has to be made between the congenitally deaf and those acquiring deafness in the post-linguistic period. The time of onset is crucial. Children with post-lingual deafness suffer surprisingly little language deficit although their language tends to become less elaborate and sophisticated with time. When the deafness is acquired soon after language has begun, lack of comprehension inevitably leads to poor vocabulary and alters articulation and voice quality (Freeman & Blockberger 1987) but, if intelligence is normal and the loss mild, few language and spelling problems can be expected.

The relationship of language development to middle ear disease is controversial (Rapin 1979, Hall & Hill 1986, Downs 1985) but children with bilateral otitis media on follow-up two years later had poor language, articulation and reading skills (Chalmers et al 1989). Children with bilateral glue ears and hearing losses had significantly lower comprehension, expressive language and auditory discrimination compared with children with no hearing losses. Their language was immature but not deviant and a rapid recovery of hearing and language followed grommet insertion (Pollak & Thomas 1992).

Children with high frequency deafness have been little studied, probably because they are often missed or misdiagnosed, being thought to suffer from a language disorder. Their expression is abnormal, with a characteristic strange voice which is recognisable when heard a few times. Phonation is odd, they make errors but symbolic language is excellent and in my experience, their language is not deviant. They learn to lipread early and are highly sensitive interpreters of gesture and touch (Chess & Korn 1971).

Language and blindness

These children have a severe linguistic deficit. Development is initially normal (Warren 1977), falling off at about 3–4 months of age when gesturing and child–mother signalling becomes delayed (Fraiburg 1977). Their linguistic behaviour is of interest as it casts light upon the visual input required for good language acquisition. Echolalia, a normal stage in language development (Cantwell et al 1978) is retained longer than average (Dyer et al 1981); symbolic language is delayed and may remain poor; the use of 'I' and 'You' may be delayed (Howlin 1980) and coding and classification of objects is late (Andersen et al 1984). The delays improve with age if the children are intelligent and may be normal by age 6–7 years (Reynell & Zinkin 1979). Blind children have special auditory skills. They are very good at role playing with voice, play games using different voices with ease, are good imitators, mimics and rhymers (Rogow 1982). Usually extremely vocal, they use their voices to gain attention and to gauge distances (Unwin 1984).

Some parents of blind or partially sighted children find the interpretation of nonverbal communication difficult because the children have 'flat' expressionless faces, smile inappropriately, stay unusually still and have a 'broadcasting' type of voice which may be due to an inability to judge the distance they are away from their audience (Jan et al 1977). A very small minority of blind children have been described as autistic-like (Fay & Schuler 1980) usually in association with retrolental fibroplasia (Chase 1972). But one might feel it was the continued use of echolalia, the absence of a recognition of gender and some grammatical errors which lead to this erroneous diagnosis. The children did not have true 'Kanner' type autism.

Blindness with deafness

Fortunately children are rarely blind-deaf. This is an awesome problem. It is usually impossible to gauge whether there is overlying severe mental retardation or the handicap is so overwhelming that communication is impossible but McInnes et al (1982) have described some techiques of observing the behaviour of such children. In an acquired case, due to progressive muscular atrophy in an older child, the visual impairment proved the greater handicap.

Certain medical conditions have an accompanying hearing or visual impairment and the combination may compound the language deficit. For example, there is a higher than expected incidence of deafness in mental retardation from ANY cause and some infections and syndromes (see Ch. 12).

Severe environmental deprivation

The Wild Boy of Aveyron and others mentioned at the beginning of this chapter are examples of extreme environmental deprivation causing lack of language development. It has been questioned (Howlin 1980) whether such children are not autistic, thus explaining their lack of language, and abandoned for this reason. However, reading the original descriptions of the Wild Boy and the Wolf children this appears extremely unlikely. If there is a sensitive period during which language needs to be acquired and which, if passed, prevents its acquisition, the histories of the Wild Boy and the Wolf children give credence to this theory; but Howlin (1980) draws attention to Genie (Curtiss 1977) who was not rescued until the age of 14 years, yet subsequently developed reasonable language despite subtle sentences remaining lacking. Caspar Hauser (Wassermann 1908) is another example. The lower language level of some children in institutions has been discussed and the amount of verbal interaction experienced rather than the institution itself is the essential ingredient (Tizard et al 1972). The language of 3-year-old Kibbutzim children was not different to a control group of Jewish children living at home (Pollak 1989).

LANGUAGE AND ASSOCIATED MEDICAL CONDITIONS

Mental retardation

Whether of known or unknown aetiology, mental retardation is the most common reason for poor language skills. One-third of the Waltham Forest Study children whose language had not improved at 7 years of age had IQs below 85 (Stevenson & Richman 1976), 39% in the Newcastle study (Fundudis et al 1979) whilst 31% of children with continued poor language skills in the Dunedin Studies had IQs below 90. All found an association between low IQ at 7 years and learning and behavioural problems. The language of mentally handicapped children is inadequate due to poor vocabulary and knowledge of words rather than deficient grammar (Spreen 1965).

Cerebral palsy

A high proportion of children with cerebral palsy have speech defects and estimates have included: 50% (Ingram 1964); 70% (Dunsden 1952) and

approximately 4.0 per 10 000 children (Lotter 1966, Wing & Gould 1979, Gillberg 1984) so it is a very rare condition. Given this rarity and if, in addition, many cases are not 'pure' but so-called 'partial' cases (Wing & Gould 1979), others not truly fitting into 'Kanner autism', the confusion surrounding autism is perhaps not surprising. When high-functioning autistic children were compared with children with Asperger syndrome it was concluded that the latter should be considered a mild form of high-functioning autism (Szatmari et al 1989). A further difficulty is that autism has been associated with all the following conditions:

Mental retardation (Clark & Rutter 1979)
Epilepsy (Ohlsson et al 1988)
Fragile X (Wahlstrom et al 1986)
Other sex chromosome abnormalities
Tuberose sclerosis (Lotter 1974)
PKT
Phenylketonuria (Friedman 1969)
Several infections, e.g rubella, herpes, cytomegalovirus (Chess et al 1971, De Long et al 1981, Stubbs et al 1984)
Moebius syndrome (Myerson & Frushee 1978)
Rett syndrome (Witt-Engerstrom & Gillberg 1987)
Lactic acidosis and purine disorders (Coleman et al 1976)
Hydrocephalus (Schain & Yannet 1960)
Duchenne muscular dystrophy (Komoto et al 1984)
Cornelia de Lange syndrome
Asperger syndrome (Tantam 1988)
Schizophrenia (Wolff & Barlow 1979, Ritvo 1977)
Neurofibromatosis (Riikonen & Amnell 1981)
Some prenatal risk factors (Finegan & Quarrington 1979)
Williams syndrome

The most practical solution is to describe the common communication abnormalities which occur in autism but it will be impossible, in addition, not to describe the abnormalities of behaviour and social development with which they are associated. Whether it is academic or there is a real need to differentiate autism as a separate entity depends on whether the therapy of autism needs to be so very different from, for example, that of severe language disorders. This will be discussed later.

Social and behavioural abnormalities associated with autism. From the earliest days, there is a lack of understanding of gesture, facial expression and feelings (Landry et al 1988). Babies do not like to be nor put up arms to be picked up. Apart from not understanding the gestures of others, they show little facial expression, cry and smile rarely and often inappropriately. Older children have gaze aversion more marked towards other children than to known adults. Autistic children do not like people and prefer inanimate objects. So, as well as gaze aversion, there is less attention seeking. They rarely initiate interaction and show a lack of the joint attention so necessary for verbal or linguistic communication (Landry & Loveland 1988). Behaviour towards play and toys is abnormal, repetitive, ritualistic behaviour and mannerisms often affecting play with toys which they often line up obsessively. Change is resisted; exactly similar routines are insisted upon which can spill over into attitudes towards toys. They become upset and aggressive if the lines are moved and there may be abnormal attachments to a toy (never a doll or cuddly toy) or object from which they will not be parted. They cannot play with but may play alongside other children. They have no friends and are socially isolated children. Abelson (1981) noted the delay or virtual absence of gender identity. Mannerisms, such as the flapping of arms, holding outstretched fingers against the light and twirling the body are seen. A complete disregard for danger and apparent lack of judgement of distance such as jumping off the top of cupboards is seen. Although non-verbal skills exceed verbal they are less good on matching tasks (Dads et al 1988) and inferior on a conditional matching learning task compared with normal and mentally retarded children of similar mental age (Prior 1977).

Generally it is believed that autistic children have normal nonverbal IQs but Graham (1986) states that only 5% have nonverbal IQs over 100; 70% being below 70 and 50% below 50. Autistic and schizophrenic children scored highest in the performance, block design and object assembly tests of the WISC (Asarnow et al 1987). 'Islets' of special skills such as rote learning or mathematical skills have been described (O'Connor & Hermelin 1984).

Language and communication problems. Severely affected children may be mute but not the majority who have some speech by 4 years of age. Speech and communication are extremely abnormal.

Early communication. A characteristic of autistic children is a failure or complete lack of preverbal skills, with no understanding of gestures, facial expression and, in older children, feelings of other people. Echolalia, a transient feature of normal language development, is retained long after 20 months of age (Dyer & Hadden 1981). Initially of the immediate type, in older children it becomes of the delayed kind, often egocentric and inappropriate (Shapiro & Huebner 1976). Toddlers will often take a carer by the hand drawing them to a desired object. Direct questions can help the child to makes his needs and wants understood.

Comprehension. Autistic children have inferior auditory discrimination and make poor functional use of language. They seem unable to extract concepts from heard language and, in older children, this leads to a conceptual deficit. These are grave language deficits.

Expression. Severe problems in comprehension inevitably lead to problems of expressive speech which is limited and may be sporadic: some children have spoken and then remained mute for several months. Syntax is primitive, articulation poor but grammar may be correct. 'I' and 'You' may be reversed and related to lack of understanding gender. Pronouns are little used. Phraseology and morphology are similar to that of specific language disordered children.

Symbolic language. Symbolic language may be entirely absent or highly abnormal (Wing et al 1977). Abnormal play has already been mentioned. Cars, often an obsession, will have wheels spun endlessly. The dearth of symbolic language and thought leads to an inability of labelling language and the absence of storage and retrieval in any symbolic form. Autistic children often learn to read well but are unable to understand what they read. I have written instructions which have been correctly read but not executed. An example is an autistic girl, asked to spell 'school', who wrote, perfectly spelt, from top to bottom of the page: Inner London Education Authority!

Thus the language and communication problems of autistic children include abnormality in every parameter of communication and language. Some visual aspects of life are partly understood and hence accentuated, which could explain the need to line up toys and why bedtime, eating and toileting must be undertaken with exactly the same procedures resulting in some stability and meaning to the day.

DIAGNOSIS: AVAILABLE TESTS AND THEIR INTERPRETATION

History

Special points of a linguistic history are:

- Questions of factors affecting development of language
- Preverbal development
- Linguistic opportunities the child has had
- Does the child share mother's time with other children (and/or adults)

Examination of language

Each of the four main parameters of communication and language development will be measured:

1. Comprehension: how much is understood of what is said to the child?
2. Expression: how much can he himself say?
3. Inner or symbolic language: how well can the child manipulate and reproduce information already obtained?
4. Speech production: does the child pronounce and articulate correctly?

Tests of comprehension

Reynell developmental language scales (Reynell 1969) (Also includes scales for expression.) Figure 9.3 illustrates miniatures and

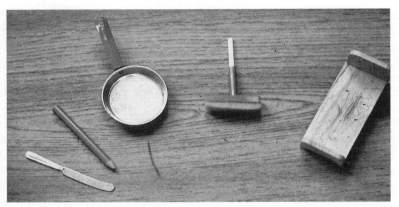

Fig. 9.3   Reynell developmental language scales.

questions which are asked are: show me the one to sleep on; cook the dinner in; sweep the floor with; write a letter and cut up the meat with. Scored for children aged 1–7 years, they are not useful for children with language ages under $1\frac{1}{2}$ years. The linguistic progression of the scales is developmentally accurate and clever use of toys matches the development in play. The tests use lifesize objects for children under 2 years and miniature toys of people, animals and objects all of which are familiar to children. Children of all ages enjoy these tests, they are reliable and useful for mentally retarded children, particularly those with Down syndrome (Rogers 1975). A language age in years and months is obtained and can be used for comparison at follow-up. There are centile charts and patients who are two or three standard deviations below the mean probably require treatment. With experience the tests are not time-consuming.

Stycar language test (Sheridan 1975) (Includes expression and symbolic language). A clinical test, this requires experience and developmental paediatric judgement — for which it has been criticized (Martlew 1978). A test of comprehension for children aged 2 years and over and young children like the materials and the social interaction between child and tester but older children may become bored. Having no age levels, it is less satisfactory as a follow-up tool.

Miniature Toys Test (Egan 1986). Includes expression and symbolic language; it can be used over the age range 18 months to 4.06 years. A modified version of the Stycar test it has the advantage of having been standardized. The word recognition and understanding of prepositions are excellent but a distinction between 'self-related' and 'detached-from-self' play is made. Unfortunately the time at which this developmental progress is made differs for different toys, making this less satisfactory.

Test for reception of grammar (TROG) (Bishop 1977) (Fig. 9.4).

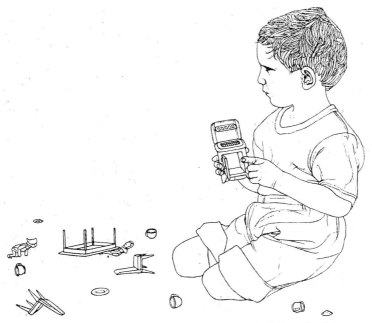

Fig. 9.6 Mentally retarded boy unable to play meaningfully with miniature toys.

Table 9.1 illustrates the complexity of elucidating comprehension. If hearing and nonverbal IQ are satisfactory, linguistic opportunities have been normal yet comprehension is lower than age, then a *developmental language problem* is most likely.

In some cases of severe language disorder and autism it is difficult to establish nonverbal skills but most children enjoy puzzles and formboards although not drawing. If the child's language development is less than two-thirds performance skill a significant language handicap exists (Sonksen 1977). Two standard deviations below the mean on Reynell scales is a useful level for a diagnosis of a serious language problem.

Table 9.1 Factors that affect the comprehension of language

	Comprehension	
	Good	Poor
Hearing	Satisfactory	Indistinct
Auditory discrimination	Well established	Listening not established
Intelligence	Average	Below average
Linguistic experience	Average	Limited

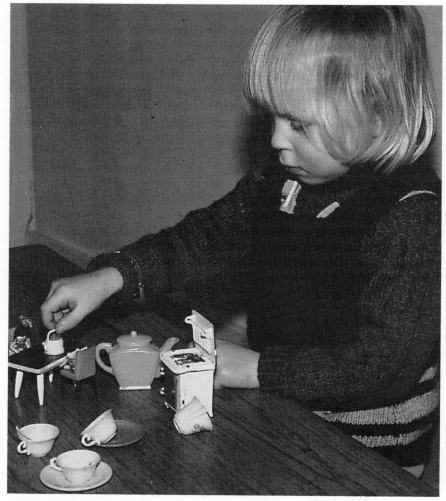

Fig. 9.7 Intelligent deaf 3-year-old with good symbolic language.

Expressive language

Expressive language is a mixture of:

- structural production of speech
- neurological intactness
- cerebral function
- adequate perception
- environmental experience.

Signing languages

Teachers of signing language have strong views about which is the best system (See Yule & Unwin 1987 for an excellent review). For children with good intellect and severe physical handicap the Bliss symbol system (1965) appears more suitable whilst the Makaton vocabulary (Cornforth et al 1974) seems preferable when the physical handicap is less but the cognitive function lower.

Stutterers

Speech therapists advise parents of young children to ignore the problem and avoid situations which produce the stammer. Andrews & Ingham (1972) suggested estimating both frequency and rate of stuttering and used these in initial treatment. This is followed by reading aloud and when children are proficient, they join a group and read aloud to other improving stutterers. 95% fluency was achieved by this method (Cave 1977). Intensive rather than once weekly visits were recommended.

Deaf children

Treatment is discussed in Chapter 11.

Mentally retarded children

The language of mentally retarded children is different to language delayed or disordered children. Treatment is discussed in Chapter 14.

Blind and partially sighted children

Because a blind baby is unable to pick up the visual clues of preverbal communication, he may appear unresponsive. Parents can be taught to be aware of the need and, by verbal and tactile stimulation preverbal communication can be translated into sound. Clapping is a good exercise as are songs with movements, rhymes and rhythms. The baby may cry or babble just to gain attention or make verbal contact and blind infants have to learn to judge distances and 'fix' patterns of their surroundings by sound, e.g. doorbells or clocks chiming. Movements and gestures (such as putting up arms to be picked up) which accompany talk have to be taught verbally. Blind children ask fewer questions compared with sighted children (Rogow 1980, 1982). Parents can help by role playing with everyday themes, imaginative games and story telling.

50–90% of blindness is associated with another handicap (Jan et al 1977) and usually complicates and affects the treatment of language problems. The Chomsky view of the development of language would conclude that the language of blind children is neither delayed nor deviant whilst Piagetians believe that language will be affected. We shall take a practical view. Young blind children have a disadvantage in perceptual and tactile learning compared with blindfolded sighted children of the same age (Gomuliki 1961). The language of blind children begins to lag when preverbal communication is preminent and the gap continues. By 5 years of age, however, the language of the intelligent blind child is good. Speech therapy should be concentrated over the ages 4–6 months to 4 years. Parents may need counselling and can be taught many ways in which to help their child (see above).

Language is one of the most important parameters of development. Delays and abnormalities in this development should be taken seriously as they have important long-term effects for the child, for the adult he will become and for society in general.

REFERENCES

Abelson A G 1981 The development of gender identity in the autistic child. Child: Care, Health and Development 7: 347–356

Abelson W D, Zigler E, deBlasi C L 1974 Effects of a four-year follow-through program on economically disadvantaged children. Journal of Educational Psychology 66: 756–771

Alajouanine T H, Lhermitte F 1965 Acquired aphasia in children. Brain 88: 653–662

Albery L, Enderby P 1984 Intensive speech therapy for cleft palate children. British Journal of Disorders of Communication 19: 115–124

American Psychiatric Association 1980 Diagnostic and Statistical Manual of Mental Disorders 3rd edn. American Psychology Association, Washington

Andersen E S, Dunlea A, Kekelis L S 1984 Blind children's language: resolving some differences. Journal of Child Language 11: 645–664

Anderson D E, Coleman R 1980 Language enhancement in the developmentally delayed child through a cognitive/receptive mode. Child: Care, Health and Development 6: 35–46

Andrews G, Harris M 1964 Stammering. In: Renfrew C, Murphy K (eds) the child who does not talk. Clinics in Developmental Medicine 13. Spastics International Medical Publication/Heinemann Medical Books, London pp. 184–192

Andrews G, Ingham R 1972 An approach to the evaluation of stuttering. Journal of Speech and Hearing Research 15: 296–302

Annett M 1973 Laterality of childhood hemiplegia and the growth of speech and intelligence. Cortex 9: 4–33

Anthony B 1971 The Edinburgh Articulation Test

Aram D, Nation J E 1975 Patterns of language behaviour in children with developmental language disorders. Journal of Speech and Hearing Research 18: 229–241

Arkell J E 1983 Logos the formula: a theoretical and practical disquisition into children's learning of the English morphology. Collected Original Resources in Education 3:

Asarnow R F, Tanquay P E, Bott L, Freeman B J 1987 Patterns of intellectual functioning in non-retarded autistic and schizophrenic children. Journal of Child Psychology and Psychiatry 28: 273–280

Bak E, van Dongen H R, Arts W F, Map 1983 Developmental Medicine 25: 81–94

Barry R M, Hardcastle B 1987 Some observations on the use of electropalatography as a clinical tool in the diagnosis and treatment of articulation disorders in children. First International Symposium on Specific Speech and Language Disorders in Children. AFASK, Reading pp. 208–222

Basser L S 1962 Hemiplegia of early onset and the faculty of speech with special reference to the effects of hemispherectomy. Brain 85: 427–460

Bax M 1975 Clinical analysis of the cry. Developmental Medicine and Child Neurology 17: 799–801

Bax M 1987 Paediatric assessment of the child with a speech and language disorder. In: Yule W, Rutter M (eds) Language development and disorders. MacKeith Press, Oxford

Bax M, Hart H, Jenkins S 1980 Assessments of speech and language development in the young child. Paediatrics 63: 350–354

Bell S M, Ainsworth M D S 1972 Infant crying and maternal responsiveness. Child Development 43: 1171–1190

Bernal J 1972 Crying during the first 10 days of life and maternal responses. Developmental Medicine and Child Neurology 14: 362

Bernstein B 1975 Class, codes and control, vol 3. Routledge, London

Bishop D 1979 Comprehension in developmental language disorders. Developmental Medicine and Child Neurology 21: 225–238

Bishop D 1982 Comprehension of spoken, written and signed sentences in childhood language disorders. Journal of Child Psychology and Psychiatry and Allied Disciplines 23: 1–20

Bishop D 1985 Age of onset and outcome in 'acquired aphasia with convulsive disorder' (Landau–Kleffner Syndrome). Developmental Medicine and Child Neurology 27: 705–712

Bishop D V M 1977 Test for Reception of Grammar. NFER–Nelson, Windsor

Bishop D, Edmundson A 1987 Specific language impairment as a maturational lag: evidence from longitudinal data on language and motor development. Developmental Medicine and Child Neurology 29: 442–459

Bishop D, Rosenbloom L 1987 Childhood language disorders: classification and overview. In: Yule W, Rutter M (eds) Language development and disorders. MacKeith Press, London

Blank M, Solomon F A 1969 How shall the disadvantaged child be taught? Child Development 40: 47–61

Bliss C 1965 Semantography. Semantography Publications, Sydney

Bloodstein O 1960a The development of stuttering. 1. Changes in nine basic features. Journal of Speech Disorders: 25: 219

Bloodstein O 1960b The development of stuttering. 2. Developmental phase. Journal of Speech Disorders 25: 366

Bloom L, Lahey M 1978 Language development and language disorders. John Wiley, New York

Bluma S, Shearer M, Frohman A, Hilliard J 1976 Manual of the Portage Guide to Early Education. NFER-Nelson, Windsor

Bowman C A, Wood C E 1983 A phonological process approach to articulation treatment. Developmental Medicine and Child Neurology 26: 238

Brown B J, Lloyd H A 1975 Controlled study of children not speaking at school. Journal of the Association of Workers for Maladjusted Children 3: 49–63

Butler N R, Golding J 1986 From birth to five. Pergamon Press, Oxford

Cantwell D, Baker L 1987 Intervention strategies for developmental language disorder and developmental articulation disorder. In: Cantwell D, Baker L (eds) Developmental speech and language disorders. Guilford Press, New York

Cantwell D, Baker L, Rutter M 1978 A comparative study of infantile autism and specific developmental receptive language disorder. IV. Analysis of syntax and language function. Journal of Child Psychology and Psychiatry and Allied Disciplines 19: 351–362

Cave D 1977 Assessment and treatment of stuttering in children. Developmental Medicine and Child Neurology 19: 410–412

Cazdan C B 1974 Play with language and metalinguistic awareness. International Journal of Early Childhood 6: 12–25

Chalmers D, Stewart I, Silva P, Mulvena A 1989 Otitis media with effusion — the Dunedin study. Clinics in Developmental Medicine 108. MacKeith Press, Oxford

Chase J B 1972 Retrolental fibroplasia and autistic symptomatology. American Foundation for the Blind, New York

Chazan M, Laing A F, Bailey M S, Jones G 1980 Some of our children: the early education of children with special educational needs. Open Books, London

Chess S, Korn S J, Fernandez P B 1971 Psychiatric disorders of children with congenital rubella. Brunner-Mazel, New York

Chomsky N 1957 Syntactic structures. Mouton Publishers, The Hague

Chomsky N 1959 Review of B F Skinner's Verbal behaviour. Language 35: 26–58.

Chomsky N 1969 Language and the mind. Psychology Today 4: 1–8

Clark P, Rutter M 1979 Task difficulty and task performance in autistic children. Journal of Child Psychology and Psychiatry and Allied Disciplines 20: 271–285

Clarke A M, Clarke A D B 1976 Early experience: myth and evidence. Open Books, London

Cohen J, Mathias R, Tronick E Z, Connell D, Lyons-Ruth K 1986 Face-to-face interactions of depressed mothers and their infants. In: Tronick E, Field T (eds) Maternal depression and infant disturbance. Jossey-Bass, San Francisco, pp.31–44

Coleman M, Landgrebe M A, Landgrebe A R 1976 Purine autism: hyperuricosuria in autistic children. Does this identify a subgroup of autism? In: Coleman M (ed) The autistic syndrome. North Holland, Amsterdam, pp 183–195

Conrad R 1979 The deaf schoolchild: language and cognitive function. Harper & Row, London

Cook J, Urwin S, Kelly K 1989 Preschool language intervention – a follow-up of some within-group differences. Child: Care, Health and Development 15: 381–400

Cooper J, Ferry P C 1978 Acquired auditory verbal agnosia and seizures in childhood. Journal of Speech and Hearing Disorders 43: 176–184

Cooper J, Moodley M, Reynell J 1979 The developmental language programme results from a five-year study. British Journal of Disorders of Communication 14: 57–69

Cornforth A R T, Johnson K, Walker M 1974 The Makaton Vocabulary. RADD, London

Costello A 1987 Preverbal communication. Journal of Child Psychology and Psychiatry and Allied Disciplines 17: 351–353

Cox A D, Puckering C, Pound A, Mills M 1987 The impact of maternal depression in young children. Journal of Child Psychology and Psychiatry and Allied Disciplines 28: 917–928

Critchley E 1967 Language development of hearing children in a deaf environment. Developmental Medicine and Child Neurology 9: 274–280

Crome L C, Stern J 1967 The pathology of mental retardation. Churchill Livingstone, Edinburgh

Cromer R F 1978 The basis of childhood dysphasia: a linguistic approach. In: Wyke M (ed) Developmental Dysphasia. Academic Press, London

Curtiss S 1977 Genie: a psycholinguistic study of a modern-day wild child. Academic Press, New York

Dadds M, Schwartz S, Adams T, Rose S 1988 The effects of social context and verbal skill on the stereotypic and task-involved behaviour of autistic children. Journal of Child Psychology and Psychiatry and Allied Disciplines 29.5: 669–676

Darley F, Aronson A, Brown J R 1969 Differential diagnostic patterns of dysarthria. Journal of Hearing Research 12: 246–269

Davie C E, Butler N, Goldstein H 1972 From birth to seven: a report of the National Child Development Study. Longman, London

Davis K 1947 Final note on a case of extreme isolation. American Journal of Sociology 45: 554–565

Delong G R, Beau S C, Brown F R 1981 Acquired reversible autistic syndrome in acute encephalopathic illness in children. Archives of Neurology 38: 191–194

Dixon J, Kot A, Law J 1988 Early language screening in City and Hackney: work in progress. Child: Care, Health and Development 14: 213–229

Douglas J E, Sutton A 1978 The development of speech and mental processes in a pair of twins: a case study. Journal of Child Psychology and Psychiatry and Allied Disciplines 19.1: 49–56

Douglas J E, Sutton A 1978 The development of speech and mental processes in a pair of twins: a case study. Journal of Child Psychology and Psychiatry and Allied Disciplines 19: 49–57

Douglas J W B 1964 The Home and the School. MacGibbon Kee, London

Downs M 1985 Identification of language delay from recurrent otitis media. Proceedings of the International Conference on Acute and Secretory Otitis Media. Kluwer, Amsterdam, pp 375–377

Dubowitz V 1965 Intellectual impairment in muscular dystrophy. Archives of Disease in Childhood 40: 296–301

Dunn J, Wooding C, Hermann J 1977 Developmental Medicine and Child Neurology 19: 629–638

Dunn L M, Dunn L M 1981 Peabody Picture Vocabulary Test – Revised. American Guidance Services, Minnesota

Dunn L M, Dunn L M, Whetton C, Pintilie D 1983 The British Picture Vocabulary Scale. NFER–Nelson, Windsor

Dunsden M I 1952 The educability of cerebral palsied children. Newnes Educational, London

Dyer C, Hadden A J 1976 A multi-axial classification for the education of autistic children. Child: Care, Health and Development 2: 155–165

Dyer C, Hadden A J 1981 Delayed echolalia in autism: some observations on differences within the term. Child: Care, Health and Development 7: 331–345

Egan D F 1986 Developmental assessment: 18 months to 4.6 years. The Miniature Toys Test. Child: Care Health and Development 12: 167–181

Fay W H, Schuler A L 1980 Emerging language in autistic children. University Park Press, Baltimore

Feitelson D 1972 Developing imaginative play in pre-school children as a possible approach to fostering creativity. Early Child Development and Care 1: 181–197

Fenn G 1976 Against verbal enrichment. In: Berry P (ed) Language and communication in the mentally handicapped. Edward Arnold, London

Finegan J, Quarrington B 1979 Pre-, peri- and neonatal factors and infantile autism. Journal of Child Psychology and Psychiatry and Allied Disciplines 20: 119–126

Floyer E B 1955 A psychological study of a city's cerebral palsied children. British Council for the Welfare of Spastics, London

Folsten S, Rutter M 1977 Infantile autism: a genetic study of 21 twin pairs. Journal of Child Psychology and Psychiatry and Allied Disciplines 18: 297–321

Fraiberg S 1977 Insights from the blind: comparative studies of blind and sighted infants. Basic Books, New York

Fraser W 1978 Speech and language development of children with Down's syndrome. Developmental Medicine and Child Neurology 20: 106–108

Freeman R, Blockberger S 1987 Language development and sensory disorder: visual and hearing impairments. In: Yule W, Rutter M (eds) Language development and disorders. MacKeith Press, Oxford

Friedman E 1969 The autistic syndrome and phenylketonuria. Schizophrenia 1: 249–261

Friedrich U, Dalby M, Staehelin-Jensen T, Brunn-Petersen G 1982 Chromosomal studies of children with developmental retardation. Developmental Medicine and Child Neurology 24: 645–652

Fundudis T, Kolvin I, Garside R F 1979 Speech-retarded and deaf children: their psychological development. Academic Press, London

Furth H G 1966 Thinking without language: psychological implications of deafness. Free Press, New York

Furth H G, Youniss J 1976 Formal operations: a comparison of deaf and hearing adolescents. In: Morehead D, Morehead A (eds) Normal and deficient child language. University Park Press, Baltimore

Genesee F 1987 Learning through two languages: studies of immersion and bilingual education. Newbury House, Cambridge, Massachusetts

Gillberg C 1984 Infantile autism and other childhood psychoses in a Swedish urban region: epidemiological aspects. Journal of Child Psychology and Psychiatry and Allied Disciplines 25: 35–43

Gillberg C 1988 The neurobiology of infantile autism. Journal of Child Psychology and Psychiatry and Allied Disciplines 29: 257–266

Gillberg C, Ohlson V, Wahlstrom J, Steffenberg S, Blix K 1988 Monzygotic female twins with autism and the fragile-X syndrome (Afrax). Journal of Child Psychology and Psychiatry and Allied Disciplines 4: 447–451

Glenn S M, Cunningham C C 1982 Recognition of the familiar words of nursery rhymes by handicapped and non-handicapped infants. Journal of Child Psychology and Psychiatry and Allied Disciplines 23: 319–327

Glenn S M, Cunningham C C, Joyce P F 1981 A study of auditory preferences in non-handicapped infants and infants with Down's syndrome. Child Development

Goldman R, Fristoe M 1969 Test of Articulation. American Guidance Services, Minnesota

Goodstein L D 1968 Psychosocial aspects of cleft palate. In: Spriestersbach D, Sherman D (eds) Cleft palate and communication. Academic Press, New York

Gordon N 1990 Acquired aphasia in childhood: the Landau–Kleffner syndrome. Developmental Medicine and Child Neurology 32: 267–274

Gorlin R J, Pindborg J J, Cohen M M 1976 Syndromes of the head and neck. McGraw-Hill, New York

Graham P 1986 Infantile autism. In: Graham P (ed) Child psychiatry: a developmental approach. Oxford Medical, Oxford p 129

Guttman E 1942 Aphasia in children. Brain 65: 205–219

Hall D M B, Hill P 1986 When does secretory otitis media affect language development? Archives of Disease in Childhood 61: 42–47

Hardcastle W J, Morgan Barry R A, Clark C J 1987 The use of instrumental phonetic procedures in assessment and remediation. In: Stengelhofen J (ed) Cleft palate: case studies in the treatment of communication disorders. Churchill Livingstone, Edinburgh

Hawkins P R 1969 Social class: the nominal group and references. Language and Speech 12: 125–135

Hewison J, Tizard J 1980 Parental involvement and reading attainment. British Journal of Educational Psychology 50: 209–215

Honig C A 1967 The treatment of velopharyngeal insufficiency palatal repair. Archivum Chirurgicum Nederlandicum 19: 71–81

Horn D G, Lorch E P, Lorch R F, Culatta B 1985 Distractibility and vocabulary deficits in children with spina bifida and hydrocephalus. Developmental Medicine and Child Neurology 27: 713–720

Howlin P 1980 Language. In: Rutter M (ed) Scientific foundations of developmental psychology. Heinemann, London

Howlin P 1987 Behaviour approaches to language training. In: Yule W, Rutter M (eds) Language development and disorders. MacKeith Press, Oxford

Howlin P, Rutter M 1987 The consequences of language delay for other aspects of development. In: Yule W, Rutter M (eds) Language development and disorders. MacKeith Press, Oxford

Illingworth R S 1970 Mental subnormality with physical defects and disease. In: The development of the infant and young child, 4th edn. Churchill Livingstone, Edinburgh

Illingworth R S 1987 The development of the infant and young child: normal and abnormal, 9th edn. Churchill Livingstone, Edinburgh

Ingram T T S 1964 Paediatric aspects of cerebral palsy. E & S Livingstone, Edinburgh

Ingram T T S 1972 The classification of speech and language disorders in young children. In: Rutter M, Martin J A M (Eds) The child with delayed speech. Clinics in Developmental Medicine 43. Spastics International Medical Publishers/Heinemann Medical Books, London

Jan J E, Freeman R D, Scott E 1977 Visual impairment in children and adolescents. Grune & Stratton, New York

Jenkins S, Bax M, Hart H 1980 Behaviour problems in pre-school children. Journal of Child Psychology and Psychiatry and Allied Disciplines 21: 5–17

Johnson W 1959 The onset of stuttering: research findings and implications. University of Minnesota Press, Minnesota

Jones R K 1966 Observations on stammering after localised cerebral injury. Journal of Neurology, Neurosurgery and Psychiatry 29: 192–195

Jones R S P 1988 Treating high-rate stereotyped behaviours in children. Child: Care, Health and Development 14.3: 175–189

Kaplan C, Osborne P, Elias E 1986 The diagnosis of muscular dystrophy in patients referred for language delay. Journal of Child Psychology and Psychiatry and Allied Disciplines 27: 545–549

Kaplan L, Elias E R 1986 Diagnosis of muscular dystrophy in patients referred for evaluation of speech. Developmental Medicine and Child Neurology 28: 110

Keeney T J, Smith N D 1971 Young children's imitation and comprehension of sentential singularity and plurality. Language and Speech 14: 373–382

Tantam D 1988 Asperger's syndrome. Journal of Child Psychology and Psychiatry and Allied Disciplines 29: 245–255

Tizard B, Cooperman O, Joseph A, Tizard J 1972 Environmental effects on language development: a study of young children in long-stay residential nurseries. Child Development 43: 337–358

Tizard B, Philps J, Plewis I 1976 Play in pre-school centres. 1. Play measures and their relation to age, sex and I.Q. 2. Effects on play of the child's social class and of the educational orientation of the centre. Journal of Child Psychology and Psychiatry and Allied Disciplines 17:251–274

Turton L J 1974 Discussion summary: early language intervention. In: Schiefelbusch R L, Lloyds L L (eds) Language perspectives: acquisition, retardation and intervention. Macmillan, London

Urwin C 1984 Communication in infancy and the emergence of language in blind children. In: Schiefelbusch R, Pickar J (eds) The acquisition of communicative competence. University Park Press, Baltimore, pp 479–524

Urwin S, Cook J, Kelly K 1988 Preschool language intervention — a follow-up study. Child: Care, Health and Development 14: 27–146

Van Harskamp F, van Dongen H R 1977 Construction and validation of different short forms of the Token Test. Neuropyschologia 15: 467–470

Van Hout A, Evrard P H, Lyon G 1985 On the positive seminology of acquired aphasia in children. Developmental Medicine and Child Neurology 27: 231–241

Wahlstrom J, Gillberg C, Gustavson K G, Holmgren B 1986 Infantile autism and the Fragile X syndrome: a Swedish population multicenter study. American Journal of Medical Genetics 23: 403–408

Warren D H 1977 Blindness and early childhood development. American Foundation for the Blind, New York

Wassermann J 1983 Caspar Hauser oder die Trägheit der Herzens. Deutsche Taschenbuch Verlag GmbH & Co., Munich

Wasz-Hockert O, Lind J, Vuorenkoski V, Partanen E, Valanne E 1968 The infant cry: a spectrographic and auditory analysis. Clinics in Developmental Medicine 30. Spastics International Medical Publications/Heinemann Medical Books, London

White M 1972 An experimental class for language disordered children. In: Rutter M, Martin J A (eds) The Child with Delayed Speech. Clinics in Developmental Medicine 42. Spastics International Medical Publications/Heinemann Medical Books, London

White M, East K 1983 The Wessex Revised Portage Language Check List. NFER-Nelson, Windsor

Williams J C, Barratt-Boyes B G, Lowe J B 1961 Supravalvular aortic stenosis. Circulation 24: 1311–1318

Wing L, Gould J 1979 Severe impairments of social interaction and associated abnormalities in children: epidemiology and classification. Journal of Autism and Developmental Disorders 9: 11–29

Wing L, Gould J, Yeates S, Brierley L 1977 Symbolic play in severely mentally retarded and autistic children. Journal of Child Psychology and Psychiatry and Allied Disciplines 18: 167–179

Witt-Engerstrom I, Gillberg C 1987 Autism and Rett syndrome: a preliminary epidemiological study of diagnostic overlap. Journal of Autism and Developmental Disorders 17: 149–150

Wolff P H 1969 The natural history of crying and other vocalisations in early infancy. In: Foss B M (ed) Determinants of infant behaviour, vol 4. Methuen, London, pp 81–109

Wolff S, Barlow A 1979 Schizoid personality in childhood: a comparative study of schizoid, autistic and normal children. Journal of Child Psychology and Psychiatry and Allied Disciplines 20: 29–46

Woods B T, Carey S 1979 Language deficits after apparent clinical recovery from childhood aphasia. Annals of Neurology 6: 405–409

Yule W, Berger M 1972 Behaviour modification principles and speech delay. In: Rutter M, Martin J A (eds) The child with delayed speech. Clinics in Developmental Medicine 43. Spastics International Medical Publications/Heinemann Medical Books, London

Yule W, Rutter M (eds) 1987 Language development and disorders. Clinics in Developmental Medicine 101/102 MacKeith Press with Heinemann Medical Books, Oxford
Yule W, Unwin O 1987 The role and value of augmented communication. First International Symposium on Specific Speech and Language Disorders in Children. AFASIC, Reading, pp 314–325

10. Play and learning

Man shall not live by bread alone

St. Matthew, Chapter 4. Verse 4.

Man needs not only food, water and shelter in order to survive; he needs to think, to know how to do things and the likely outcome of events. Learning is therefore no luxury — although it can be a most pleasurable activity.

The skills which enable man to adapt to his environment are often regarded as a measure of his intelligence but most are far removed from the average test of intelligence. The brain is the organ of learning and, just as the brain goes through developmental stages, so too, does learning.

PIAGETIAN THEORY

We owe much of our knowledge of learning processes to the work of Jean Piaget (1896–1979) whose life's work was a study of the stages through which children's thinking and learning progress and a summary is:

Basic principles

1. Every baby is born with strategies for interacting with his environment, e.g. seeing, hearing, touching, sucking, smelling and grasping.
2. Primitive strategies become modified, refined, enlarged as a result of experience of the environment.
3. Reactions to events, initially automatic, become explorative and purposeful.

All go through developmental sequences.

Stages of reaction

The process by which these sophistications of reaction take place is through:

Assimilation — 'taking in' and adapting experiences.

Accommodation — reactions are modified in the light of experience, tempered by the baby's improving powers of understanding.
Schemata — strategies or action patterns which babies and children believe are appropriate and are the result of assimilation and accommodation.

Piaget described four stages in the development of thinking:

Sensorimotor stage (birth to 2 years)

0–1 month:	almost entirely reflex.
1–4 months:	visual, auditory and tactile experiments with body.
4–10 months:	tries to repeat happenings and develops object concept.
10–12 months:	combines actions into strategies.
12–18 months:	definitely experiments to produce new situations.
18–24 months:	beginning of 'internal representation' or symbolism.

Preoperational thought (2–6 years)

The thought of the preschool child has certain characteristics: it is *egocentric*. At 2 years the child can only see things 'through his own eyes' and has to 'decentralize' his thinking and understanding. It is *simple* in that he begins his second year with primitive reasoning which can only hold one idea at a time but by 6 years old he learns to understand more than one idea or concept at a time and to deduce by using reasoning rather than association.

Concrete operational thought (6–12 years)

The child is now able to use 'learned' concepts or internal schemes which Piaget called *operations*. Some schemes are intellectual ideas learned from language and adaptive development. The child can apply these skills to school learning tasks.

Formal operational thought (12 years upwards)

The child can use deductive logic and systematic problem solving, the major advance being the conceptualization of ideas and the ability to reason with abstract thoughts and ideas outside current experience.

There are criticisms, adaptations and alterations of Piaget's work. The main criticisms are:

- Piaget underestimated children's achievements in some areas.
- Children's learning is more influenced by social and cultural environmental experiences than Piaget believed (Bruner 1973).

- Children are different and not all children conform to Piaget's stages of development.
- Differing views are held on the influence which language exerts in the development of thoughts.

Piaget's view was that thinking arises out of action; language is a symbolic aid to thought as is reading. Thought is first and language second. Others believe that language arises de novo and therefore thought arises from language (e.g. Vygotskii 1976, Chomsky 1965). It is rather important which of these theories is correct.

Despite criticisms the main bulk of Piaget's work remains seminal and is the classical foundation on which further additions and amendments are made.

For practical purposes, learning is divided into:

— learning which is an intrinsic biological attribute
— learning which is 'man-made'.

Doubtless the latter depends upon biological mental processes in order to be acquired but the three 'Rs' are man-made in the sense that it is extremely unlikely that the average child would acquire them without being taught. Drawing his daddy he might manage but writing his name he would not. It is postulated that some mental operations are innately automatic and do not undergo development, i.e. they are equal in young and old and unaffected by practice, motivation and arousal whilst other mental processes are nonautomatic and need conscious controlled effort, i.e. attention and understanding (Hasher & Zacks 1979) and possibly 'man-made' learning comes into the latter category. The acquisition of reading, writing and spelling assumes the intrinsic biological attributes have developed almost to maturity and these, together with attention and understanding, make learning the three 'Rs' possible. The development of the alphabet is the final crucial sequence in the simplification and phoneticization of writing, i.e. the basic unit of writing is a pure phonetic sign and development of writing is distinguished by increasing phoneticization and simplification (Russell 1982).

Methods of learning

Observation and listening

Three different centuries and locations illustrate timeless methods of learning which psychologists call 'learning modelling'. In Figure 10.1, Federico de Montefeltro is reading to his eldest son in Urbino (15th century). Figure 10.2 shows Pieter de Hooch's little girl in Holland watching her mother (17th century), and in Figure 10.3 the little boy in Nigeria is watching his grandmother (20th century).

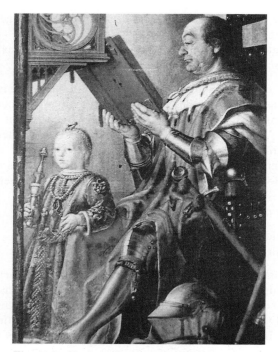

Fig. 10.1   Frederico de Montefeltro reading to his eldest son, 15th century (From *Frederico de Montefeltro con il figlio Guidubaldo* by Pietro Berruguete, courtesy of the Museo de Pallazzo, Urbino).

Imitation

Trying out what others do is a favourite method of learning and has all the hallmarks of a learning process: observation, adaptation and reproduction, i.e. assimilation, accommodation and production of a schemata (Fig. 10.4). It could be said that Wolfgang Mozart has assimilated and accommodated what father Leopold showed him. He certainly developed schemata!

Conditioning

Behaviour can be altered and learning takes place by conditioning. This is the classical learning theory: a baby is touched on the cheek, turns to the touch and begins to suck. This is an unconditioned stimulus producing an unconditioned response but if a new element is introduced, (e.g. before the above sequence of events the baby is always picked up from his cot) he can 'learn' to turn and suck without the touching prompt. The sucking has become a conditioned response to a conditioned stimulus. Learning can be induced by operant conditioning by the use of positive and negative reinforcements.

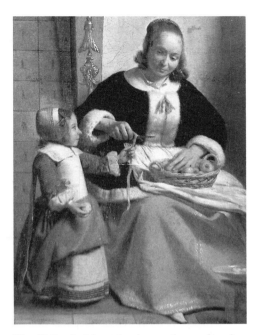

Fig. 10.2   A girl watches her mother peel apples, 17th century (Pieter de Hooch, courtesy of The Wallace Collection).

Development of thought

Young babies cannot imagine an existence separate from themselves and do not recognize that natural phenomena are alive — living creatures with feelings and actions of their own. Later they learn there are creatures other than themselves but give feelings and thoughts to animals and phenomena, e.g. 'The rain was naughty'. Eventually, natural phenomena and inert material are recognized as being without feelings. *The newborn baby* can root and suck if a object is placed near his mouth but cannot distinguish the nipple or teat from a finger or pencil. He reacts to all four in the same way. *By the first few weeks of life,* a baby 'habituates' to repetitions of the same stimuli, becomes 'bored' and searches for new, different stimuli. Whether this is true learning or not it certainly is an early manifestation of that natural curiosity which is all-important to the development of man. The new baby reacts to bright lights, sudden noises or movements, smell and taste. Initially involuntary reflex actions, they become more and more under his voluntary control. *By 6–8 months* he has learnt one of the first tasks, making his own reaction to an event — a reaction which he repeats until he can reproduce it at will (e.g. peek-a-boo).

Initially, he can only react to one thing at a time, and has only one

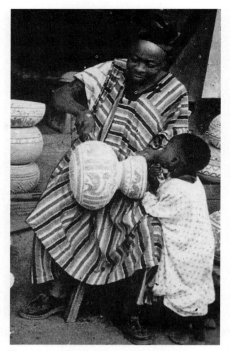

Fig. 10.3   Boy in Nigeria watching his grandmother making pottery, 20th century.

reaction but reactions become more complex and diverse as experience and cognitive powers increase. At *12–18 months* he experiments to see what will result from a different reaction and by *18–24 months* he can symbolize, which is the beginning of serious thinking and concepts. This ability will eventually lead to the conceptualization of ideas, logical thought and, through the use of symbols, to writing, reading and mathematics. By the *end of 3 years,* higher mental processes such as thinking, perceiving and understanding — the cognitive abilities — allow the child to begin to categorize, interpret and store observed information.

Development of concepts of shape and size

The development of *shape* recognition is described in more detail in Chapter 8. *By 2 days of age* he prefers to follow stripes rather than a solid colour. *By 4 months* he knows object constancy. *By 18–20 months* he recognizes a round shape, by *3 years* recognizes a square and triangle and by *5 years* knows many shapes but not yet left and right which may lead to inaccurate descriptions.

He will learn *size.* At *18 months* he does not understand one object is bigger than another but by $2\frac{1}{2}$ *years* understands bigger and smaller

(Newsom & Newsom 1979). Holt (1975) builds a compelling case for enrichment programmes for handicapped children advocating starting programmes as soon as possible. Those who devise these programmes need a sound knowledge of child development and play.

Culture

Play has a long history — marbles were a favourite sport in ancient Egypt. Play has been defined as lacking a purpose but we can agree that play represents children's work (Sheridan 1977, Chess et al 1965). Opie & Opie (1969) saw play as serving both social and individual functions. In some countries and ethnic groups there is no tradition of toys and play and in particular no symbolic play (Feitelson 1977). Children in these cultures seem to undertake work tasks as a method of learning about life. In some, child labour is a necessity (Rosenblatt 1980). Feitelson (1977) in a study of Israeli Jews from four different backgrounds, graphically describes their different patterns of play or lack of it. If play (or work) helps one to learn about life, one imagines that a 3-year-old on the banks of the Nile helping his father till the soil (Fig. 10.9); a young entrepreneur in

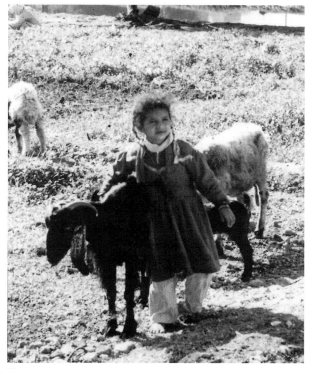

Fig. 10.9   A 3-year-old on the banks of the Nile happily helping tend the goats.

Delhi (Fig. 10.10) and a 6-year-old selling melons in Kashmir (Fig. 10.11) would learn rather more quickly than those playing with teddy bears!

Bedouin children aged 3 living in the Negev desert and Ethiopian immigrants in Israel had a lack of toys (Pollak 1981). A similar pattern was found amongst West Indians living in Brixton (Pollak 1972) and Negro Americans in South Carolina (Pollak 1979). The pattern of work (or play) was not the same amongst the four groups. Both Bedouin and Ethiopian children were busy following their mothers on her daily house-keeping round, had tasks in the preparation of food, fetching and carrying of water and even sewing and looking after even smaller siblings was common at age 3 (Fig. 10.12). The West Indian and Negro Americans were left to their own devices and had little verbal interplay with adults.

Factors which affect learning

Curiosity and attention

The natural curiosity of the human being is a requisite for learning. Attentiveness (or curiosity) is an arousal state of the mind which makes it especially receptive to particular features in the environment. One of the most striking characteristics of babies who are later found to have a very high IQ is the curiosity and powers of attention which they display in early life. Attention goes through developmental phases. There has not been as much research on attention as the subject warrants. Some facts are:

1. A *newborn baby's* attention needs to be 'caught' by a moving or bright object.

2. *By 2 months* the baby can select for himself certain objects at which to look. Although a moving and/or bright object are what initially catch attention, the baby has now learned to look and scan whole objects seemingly of his own volition. Novel objects are now of prime importance. The edges of objects are scanned. The baby is learning social attention — his mother coos and smiles at him and he learns to smile back. This, in turn, produces further reaction. He can only attend to one stimulus at a time.

3. *By 4 months* he can deal with more than one stimulus. He scans objects up and down as well as the edges. Probably the most important aspect of attention is the 'selective attention' which enables children to attend to one of many stimuli simultaneously presented to them. Not only do they learn to select but they improve in sustaining attention upon their choice. This is noticeable in young children with mental ages far in excess of chronological age. Their concentration is intense whilst it lasts but they do have the maturity to sustain the attention span of an average child with an equivalent mental age. Scanning gets increasingly complex and intricate with age and maturity.

Environmental factors

Socio-economic status

That reading and academic progress are lower in children of low socioeconomic status (SES) is well known and the evidence not reiterated. Most studies do not dissociate low SES from intelligence but one study was able to do so. 50 children aged from 5 years 8 months to 6 years 8 months, in a low socio-economic area, were matched for sex and IQ with 50 children from a middle-class area. At the later age, the former were significantly lower on reading and number concepts than the middle-class children (Bell et al 1976). The standard of mathematics in poor areas is lower than in better off districts (Barakat 1951). A variety of theories has been advanced to explain these differences: low parental expectations (Deutsch 1965); more help in middle-class homes (John 1963); fewer experiences and poorer language in homes with low SES status (Bereiter 1972); low self-esteem (Reid 1972). The vocabulary of school entrants from disadvantaged homes was adequate for starting to read but one year later children from advantaged homes were ahead of the disadvantaged children. This was considered due to the lack of books in the disadvantaged homes (Francis 1974).

Play

Children learn through play (Sheridan 1975). Thus a lack may delay learning. Play has already been discussed.

School

The problems children encountered by two successive intakes into 13 infant schools in inner London were studied. Half a term after they first started 13% were rated as having difficulty in coping with school life and learning (Hughes et al 1979). Boys encountered more problems than girls. Concentration was the problem most commonly reported (28%) whilst 25% were rated as lacking self-reliance, having difficulty in following instructions and/or having poor fine motor control. All are factors involved in the learning process. There is a high incidence of severe reading backwardness in children who are maladjusted (Chazan 1969, Chazan & Jackson 1974, Davie et al 1972). Between 14 and 23% of pupils in a deprived catchment area were judged by their teachers to be poorly adjusted with resultant learning problems (Cox 1978). By showing that characteristics which are unique to a school can affect the behaviour and achievement of its pupils, Rutter et al (1979) demonstrated the strong effect which schools can have upon children's learning. Pupil characteristics and background are not the only determinants of pupils' outcome (Reynolds 1982). Bax (1974) has been one of the few persistently advising the paediatrician to go into schools.

Medical factors

Low birthweight

The evidence is conflicting. The follow-up study of low birthweight children at school entry (Drillien et al 1980) excluded *low birthweight* per se as a cause of learning problems; problems at school being related to social class, intrauterine insult, postnatal complications and neurodevelopmental status during the first year of life. Multiple birth, gestation and intrauterine growth retardation were also not related to learning problems. However, other studies have shown that children who are *small for gestational age* have temperamental differences which may lead to learning problems (Parkinson et al 1986, 1981; Harvey et al 1982) and *preterm birth and low birthweight* were significant antecedents of poor reading, spelling and mathematics in the study of Zubrick et al (1988).

Hearing loss

Learning problems are common amongst children with severe deafness. In the study of childhood deafness in the European Community, Martin & Moore (1979) found a positive relationship between poor reading ability and severity of hearing loss. But a less severe loss or an intermittent hearing loss due to middle ear disease have not been incontrovertibly associated with school learning problems.

Vision

The following quotation from Gardiner (1974) cannot be bettered: 'Vision, visual acuity and visual skills have parts to play in learning. The visual apparatus exists to present information to be decoded and acted upon by the subject. This is the object of the whole complex. If there are defects in the transmission of the message to be decoded, then the interpretation is liable to be affected. If there are defects in those areas of the brain which perform the decoding then, however good the information, the message may be garbled. Lastly, the action which results depends upon the subject grasping the meaning, significance and implication of the information, and on his understanding that this implies a need for action'.

Chronic illness and disability

Approximately 30–40% of children who are chronically ill or handicapped suffer school related problems (Schlieper 1985). Chronically ill children are likely to have one or some factors which affect their academic learning:

1. A high absence from school
2. Stress and anxiety
3. Conditions which sap energy and determination
4. Pain.

Carroll H C M 1972 The remedial teaching of reading: an evaluation. Remedial Education 7: 10–15

Chadwick O, Rutter M, Shaffer D, Shrout P E 1981 A prospective study of children with head injuries. IV. Specific cognitive deficits. Journal of Clinical Neuropsychology 3: 101–120

Chall J 1967 Learning to read: the great debate. McGraw Hill, New York

Chazan M 1969 Maladjustment and reading difficulties: recent research and experiment. Remedial Education 4: 119–123

Chazan M, Jackson S 1974 Behaviour problems in the infant school: changes over two years. Journal of Child Psychology and Psychiatry and Allied Disciplines 15: 33–46

Chess S, Thomas A, Birch H 1965 Your child is a person. Viking Press, New York

Chomsky N 1965 Aspects of the theory of syntax. MIT Press, Cambridge, Massachusetts

Clark M M 1970 Reading difficulties in schools. Penguin Books, Harmondsworth

Clarke-Stewart K A, Van Der Stoep L P, Killian G A 1979 Analysis and replication of mother-child relations at two years of age. Child Development 50: 777–793

Cox T 1978 Children's adjustment to school over six years. Journal of Child Psychology and Psychiatry and Allied Disciplines 19: 363–371

Critchley E M R 1968 Reading retardation, dyslexia and delinquency. British Journal of Psychiatry 114: 1537–1547

Cruickshank W M 1972 Some issues facing the field of learning disabilities. Journal of Learning Disabilities 5: 380–383

Dansky J L 1980 Cognitive consequences of sociodramatic play and exploration training for economically disadvantaged preschoolers. Journal of Child Psychology and Psychiatry and Allied Disciplines 20: 47–58

Davie R, Butler N, Goldstein H 1972 From birth to seven. The second Report of the National Child Development Study (1983 cohort). Longman, London

Day J B, Wedell K 1972 Visual and auditory memory in spelling. An exploratory study. British Journal of Educational Psychology 42: 33–39

Dencker S J, Lofving B 1958 A psychometric study of identical twins discordant for close head injury. Acta Psychiatrica et Neurologica Scandinavica 33: suppl 122

Deutsch M 1965 The role of social class in language development and cognition. American Journal of Orthopsychiatry 35: 78

Dillon H, Leopold R L 1961 Children and the post-concussion syndrome. Journal of the American Medical Association 175: 86–92

Doehring D G 1968 Patterns of impairment on specific reading disability. Indiana University Press, Bloomington

Douglas J W B 1964 The home and the school. A study of ability and attainment in the primary school. MacGibbon and Kee, London

Douglas V I, Barr E G, O'Neill M E, Britton B G 1986 Short term effects of methylphenidate on the cognitive, learning and academic performance of children with attention deficit disorder in the laboratory and the classroom. Journal of Child Psychology and Psychiatry 272: 191–211

Downing J 1977 Review: the use of the initial teaching alphabet with emotionally disturbed and socially maladjust children. Child: Care, Health and Development 3: 363–372

Drillien C M, Thomson A J M, Burgoyne K 1980 Low birthweight children at early school age: a longitudinal study. Developmental Medicine and Child Neurology 22: 26–47

Dunn J, Wooding C 1977 Play in the home and it's implications for learning. In: Tizard B, Harvey D (eds) Biology of play. Heinemann Medical Books, London

Dunn L M, Dunn L M 1981 PPVT Peabody Picture Vocabulary Test—revised. Manual for forms L and M, AGS. Circle Pines, Minnesota

Durrell D D 1955 Durrell analysis of reading difficulty. Harcourt, Brace Jovanich & World, USA

Eisenberg L 1966 The epidemiology of reading retardation and a program for preventive intervention. In: Money J (ed) The disabled reader: education of the dyslexic child. Johns Hopkins Press, Baltimore

Elkind D 1971 Measuring young minds. Horizon 13: 35

Erikson E H 1955 Sex differences in the play configurations of American preadolescents. In: Mead M, Wolfestein N M (eds) Childhood in contemporary cultures. University of Chicago Press, Chicago

Feitelson D 1977 Cross cultural studies of representational play. In: Tizard B, Harvey D (eds) Biology of play. Heinemann Medical Books, London

Feitelson D, Ross G 1973 The neglected factor — play. Human Development 16: 202–223

Francis H 1974 Social background, speech and learning to read. British Journal of Educational Psychology 44: 290–299

Frostig M, Maslow P 1973 Learning problems in the classroom. Grune & Stratton, New York

Fuld P A, Fisher P 1977 Recovery of intellectual ability after closed head-injury. Developmental Medicine and Child Neurology 19: 495–502

Garai J E, Scheinfeld A 1968 Sex differences in mental and behavioural traits. Genetic and Psychology Monographs 77: 169–299

Gardiner P 1974 The eye and learning disability. Annotation. Developmental Medicine and Child Neurology 16: 95–96

Gates A I 1936 Failure in reading and social maladjustment. Journal of the National Educational Association 25: 205

Gath A, Smith M A, Baum J D 1980 Emotional, behavioural and educational disorders in diabetic children. Archives of Disease in Childhood 55: 371–375

Gibson D 1978 Down's syndrome: the psychology of mongolism. Cambridge University Press, Cambridge

Gibson E J 1969 Principles of perceptual learning and development. Appleton-Century-Crofts, New York

Gillberg I C, Gillberg C, Rasmussen P 1983 Three year follow-up at age 10 of children with minor neurodevelopmental disorders. II. School achievement problems. Developmental Medicine and Child Neurology 25: 566–573

Gittelman-Klein K, Klein D 1976 Methylphenidate effects in learning disabilities: psychometric changes. Archives of General Psychiatry 33: 655–664

Gordon N 1972 Reading retardation. Developmental Medicine and Child Neurology 14: 520–523

Gregory H 1976 The deaf child and his family. Allen & Unwin, London

Haecan H 1976 Acquired aphasia in children and the ontogenesis of hemispheric functional specialisation. Brain and Language 3: 114–134

Harlow H, McGaugh J, Thompson R 1971 Psychology. Albion, San Francisco

Hartley R 1986 Imagine you're clever. Journal of Child Psychology and Psychiatry and Allied Disciplines 27: 383–398

Harvey D, Price J, Bunton J, Parkinson C E, Campbell S 1982 Abilities of children who were small-for-gestational-age babies. Pediatrics 69: 296–300

Hasher L, Zacks R T 1984 Automatic processing of fundamental information: the case of frequency of occurrence. American Journal of Psychology 39: 1372–1388

Heiskanen O, Kaste M 1974 Late prognosis of severe brain injury in children. Developmental Medicine and Child Neurology 16: 11–14

Helms D B, Turner J S 1976 Exploring child behavior. W B Saunders, Philapelphia

Hewison J 1982 The current status of remedial intervention for children with reading problems. Developmental Medicine and Child Neurology 24: 183–193

Hier D B, Lemay M, Rosenberger P B, Perlo V P 1978 Developmental dyslexia. Archives of Neurology 35: 90–92

Hinshelwood J 1895 Word-blindness and visual memory. Lancet 2: 1564–1570

Hinshelwood J 1917 Congenital word-blindness. Lewis, London

Holmes C S, Hayford J T, Gonzales J L, Weydert J A 1983 A survey of cognitive functioning at different glucose levels in diabetic persons. Diabetes Care 6: 180–185

Holt K S 1975 The handicapped child. Child: Care, Health and Development 1: 185–189

Hooweg J, Stanfield J P 1976 The effects of protein energy malnutrition in early childhood on intellectual and motor abilities in later childhood and adolescence. Developmental Medicine and Child Neurology 18: 330–350

Hughes M, Pinkerton G, Plewis I 1979 Children's difficulties on starting infant school. Journal of Child Psychology and Psychiatry and Allied Disciplines 20: 187–196

Illingworth R S 1987 The development of the infant and young child. Churchill Livingstone, Edinburgh, p 166

Ingram T T S 1970 The nature of dyslexia. In: Young F A, Lindsley D B (eds) Early experience and visual information processing in reading disorders. National Research Council, Washington

Jersild A T 1968 Child psychology, 6th edn. Prentice Hall, Englewood Cliffs

John V P 1963 The intellectual development of slum children: some preliminary findings. American Journal of Orthopsychiatry 33: 813

Johnston C, Prior M, Hay D 1984 Prediction of reading disability in twin boys. Developmental Medicine and Child Neurology 26: 588–595

Jones B 1966 Social class and the under fives. New Society 22.12.66.935

Kahn D, Birch H G 1968 Development of auditory-visual integration and reading achievement. Perceptual and Motor Skills 27: 459–468

Karagan N J, Richman L C, Sorensen J P 1980 Analysis of verbal disability in Duchenne muscular dystrophy. Journal of Nervous and Mental Disease 168: 419–423

Keir G H 1977 Review: children with reading difficulties. Child: Care, Health and Development 3: 129–141

Kruteskii V A 1976 The psychology of mathematical abilities in schoolchildren. University of Chicago Press, Chicago

Lansdown R 1978 Retardation in mathematics: a consideration of multi-factorial determination. Journal of Child Psychology and Psychiatry and Allied Disciplines 19: 181–185

Lansdown R 1978 The learning-disabled child: early detection and prevention. Developmental Medicine and Child Neurology 20: 496–497

Lansdown R 1984 Perceptual development. Child Development: Heinemann Medical Books, London, p 114

Larsen S C, Hammill D D 1974 The relationship of selected visual-perceptual abilities to school learning. Journal of Special Education 9: 281–291

Lawson J S, Inglis J 1984 The psychometric assessment of children with learning disabilites: an index derived from a principal components analysis of the WISC-R. Journal of Learning Disabilities 17: 517–522

Lawson J S, Inglis J 1985 Learning disabilites and intelligence tests results: a model based on a principal components analysis of the WISC-R. British Journal of Psychology 76: 35–48

Leblanc A F 1969 Time orientation and time estimation. A function of age. Journal of Genetic Psychology 115: 187–194

Lehman H C, Witty P 1927 The psychology of play activities. Barnes, New York

Levy H B 1983 Developmental dyslexia — a talent deficit. Developmental Medicine and Child Neurology 25: 691–692

Liberman I Y, Shankweiler D, Fischer F W, Carter B 1974 Explicit syllable and phoneme segmentation in the young child. Journal of Expiremental Child Psychology 18: 201–212

Loiseille D L, Stamm J S, Maitiniskt S, Whipple S C 1980 Evoked potential and behavioural signs of attentive dysfunctions in hyperactive boys. Psychophysiology 17: 193–201

Lunzer E A 1959 Intellectual development in the play of young children. Education Review 11: 205

Luria A R 1963 The mentally retarded child. Macmillan, New York

Macfarlane Smith I 1964 Spatial ability. University of London Press, London

MacKeith R 1977 Do disorders of perception occur? Developmental Medicine and Child Neurology 19: 821–824

Malmquist E 1958 Factors related to reading disabilites in the first grade of elementary school. Almquist, Stockholm

Martin J A M, Moore W J 1979 Childhood deafness in the European Community. Commission of the European Communities (EUR 6413)

Martlew M 1989 Observations on a child with cerebral palsy and her twin sister made in an integrated nursery and at home. Child: Care, Health and Development 15: 175–194

McMichael P 1979 The hen or the egg? Which comes first — antisocial behaviour or reading disability. British Journal of Educational Psychology 49: 226–238

Mills M, Puckering C, Pound A, Cox A 1985 What is it about depressed mothers that influences their children's functioning? In: Stevenson J E (ed) Recent research in developmental psychopathology. Pergamon Press, Oxford, pp 11–17

Mogford K 1977 The play of handicapped children. In: Tizard B, Harvey D (eds) The biology of play. Heinemann Medical Books, London

Morgan R T T 1976 "Paired reading" tuition. A preliminary report on a technique for parental tuition of reading retarded children. Journal of Child Psychology and Psychiatry and Allied Disciplines 20: 151–160

Myklehurst H R 1973 Development of disorders of written language. Studies of normal and exceptional children. Grune & Stratton, New York

Nelson H E, Warrington E K 1974 Developmental spelling retardation and it's relation to other cognitive abilities. British Journal of Psychology 65: 265–274

Newsom J, Newsom E 1966 Rights and privileges of property and play. In: 4 years old in an urban community. Pelican, London

Newsom J, Newsom E 1979 Toys and playthings in development and remediation. Allen & Unwin, London

Newton M 1970 A neuropsychological investigation into dyslexia. In: Franklin A W, Naidoo S (eds) Assessment and teaching of dyslexic children. Invalid Children's Aid Association, London

O'Connor N O, Hermelin B 1990 The recognition failure and graphic success of idiot-savant artists. Journal of Child Psychology and Psychiatry and Allied Disciplines 31: 203–215

O'Connor N, Hermelin B 1988 Low intelligence and special abilities. Journal of Child Psychology and Psychiatry and Allied Disciplines 29.4: 391–396

O'Hare A E, Brown K 1989a Childhood dysgraphia. 2. A study of hand function. Child: Care, Health and Development 15:151–166

O'Hare A E, Brown J K 1989b Childhood dysgraphia. 1. An illustrated clinical classification. Child: Care, Health and Development 15: 79–104

Olch D 1971 Effects of hemophilia upon intellectual growth and academic achievement. Journal of Genetic Psychology 119: 63–74

Opie L, Opie P 1969 Children's games in street and playground. Oxford University Press, London

Orton S T 1937 Reading, writing and speech problems in children. Chapman and Hall, London

Osterreich P A 1944 Le test de copie d'une figure complexe. Archives of Psychology 30: 205–356

Parkinson C E, Scrivener R, Graves L, Bunton J, Harvey D 1986 Behavioural differences of school age children who were small-for-dates babies. Developmental Medicine and Child Neurology 28: 498–505

Parkinson C E, Wallis S, Harvey D 1981 School achievement and behaviour of children who were small-for-dates at birth. Developmental Medicine and Child Neurology 23: 41–50

Patel S, Bharucham E P 1972 The Bender Gestalt Test as a measure of Perceptual and visuo-motor defects in cerebral palsied children. Developmental Medicine and Child Neurology 14: 156–160

Phemister M R, Richardson A M, Thomas G V 1978 Observations of young normal and handicapped children. 4: 247–259

Phillips R 1967 Children's games. In: Sloveno R, Knight J (eds) Motivation in play, games and sports. Charlestone Thomas, Springfield

Pinkerton F, Watson D R, McCelland R J 1989 A neurophysiological study of children with reading, writing and spelling difficulties. Developmental Medicine and Child Neurology 31: 569–581

Pollak M 1972 Housing and mothering. Archives of Disease in Childhood 54: 54–58

Pollak M 1972 Today's three-year-olds in London. Heinemann Medical Books, London

Pollak M 1981 A longitudinal study of the socio-economic cultural factors in the health and development of three groups of London children. Journal of Social Medicine 10: 633–638

Pollak M 1988 Paper read at 'Together for children' — multidisciplinary conference on health, sickness and disability in childhood, Kensington, London

Pollak M 1988 Three-years-old around the World. Paper read at first International Congress of Social Paediatrics. Munich

Pollak M, Tuchler H 1982 The Pollak Tapper. Head Teachers Review, Summer: 19–20

Prior M, Frye S, Fletcher C 1987 Remediation for subgroups of retarded readers using a modified oral spelling procedure. Developmental Medicine and Child Neurology 29: 64–71

Rapoport J, Mikkelsen E 1978 Antidepressants. In: Werry J S (ed) Pediatric psychopharmacology: the use of behavior modifying drugs in children. Brunner/Mazel, New York, pp 208–233

Raven J C 1938 Progressive Matrices. Sets A, B, C, D, & E. H K Lewis, London

Reid J F 1972 Reading problems and practices. Ward Lock Educational, London

Reynolds D 1982 The search for effective schools. School Organisation 2: 215–237

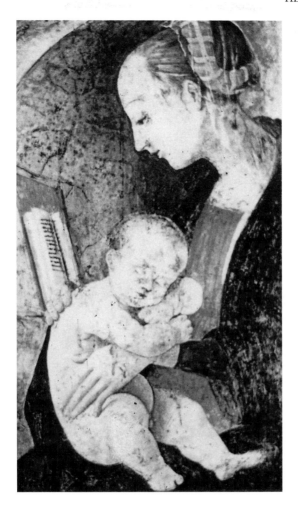

Fig. 11.9   Left ear developed in advance of the right?
(From Raffaello Sanzio Fresco *Egislente netta casa natale del pittore*, courtesy of Academic Raffaello, Urbino).

Types of hearing loss

The development of hearing involves two functions: the conduction and the perception of sound. Hence, hearing losses are divided into:

- *conductive* losses which involve the middle ear, the external meatus and tympanic membrane and
- *sensorineural* deafness which affects the cochlea, acoustic nerve and the central nervous system.

There are *mixed* types; some conductive losses are *intermittent* whilst some losses affect only certain *frequencies*. Some children with sensorineural deafness can hear only a few frequencies at normal levels, many not being heard at all, whilst other frequencies cannot be tolerated at loud decibels. The *range* of hearing is therefore very restricted and there is a problem of *recruitment*. Some sensorineural losses are *progressive*. Hearing loss may be *unilateral* or *bilateral*.

Table 11.1 shows the percentages of different types in 3000 children with hearing losses aged 8 years living in the European Communities in 1979 (Martin & Moore 1979).

The aetiology of deafness can be classified as:

- Genetic
- Prenatal (maternal)
- Perinatal
- Postnatal.

Table 11.2 shows the types of prenatal causes due to maternal problems, perinatal and postnatal causes of hearing losses respectively.

Sensorineural deafness

The majority is *congenital*. Approximately one in three deaf adults have been born deaf and over 50% of children with severe hearing losses will have suffered the loss before they were 1 year old. The majority of

Table 11.1 Percentage distribution of reported cases of childhood deafness in the European community (data from Martin & Moore 1979)

	Congenital	29%	
Genetic			9.3%
Rubella			16.7%
Other			3.2%
	Perinatal	15%	
Anoxia			5.5%
Jaundice			3.8%
Other causes			3.7%
Anoxia/jaundice			0.9%
Anoxia/other			0.6%
Jaundice/other			0.3%
Missing data			14.1%
	Acquired	14.4%	
Meningitis			7.0%
Ototoxic drugs			0.9%
Hereditary			2.0%
Other causes			4.5%
	Unknown	27.5%	
Congenital/acquired			27.5%

his/her developmental parameters and his family history require assessment. For an excellent review of syndromes associated with deafness see Konigsmark & Gorlin (1976). Fortunately, the deafblind child is a rarity. This is a disastrous combination especially since deaf children have to rely upon visual perceptive skills more than a hearing child. Many associated conditions (see Table 11.4) compound the disablement of deafness and are associated with abnormal physical appearance which only increases the feeling of alienation which many deaf children experience.

Intelligence

Intelligence and the presence of another handicap are the two factors which most affect outcome. The relationship of deafness to IQ is complex and special tests are required if the deaf child is not to be penalized on verbal aspects. There is a 'falling-off' in performance as the child grows older, so the ultimate IQ depends upon experience as well as potential. The poor communication experienced by many deaf children may be culminative and explain this 'falling-off'. Deaf children without brain damage do as well as hearing children on nonverbal tests, suggesting their nonverbal IQ (Pinter & Levy 1939, Mogford 1988, Furth & Youniss 1976, van Zyl & Ives 1971) and thought processes and sequencing skills are normal (Furth 1966, O'Connor & Hermelin 1978). Unfortunately many of the handicaps with which deaf children are associated are also associated with mental retardation, e.g. Accardo & Capute (1979) estimate approximately 15% of the deaf population are mentally retarded.

EFFECTS OF HEARING LOSS

The most important effect of deafness in children is on their language development and communication — an effect which depends upon the type, severity and time of acquisition of the deafness. The language of deaf children is discussed in Chapter 10.

Pre-linguistic language in the deaf baby

The pre-verbal language stage of the pre-linguistically deaf baby is very important as the visual element characterizes this stage (Dodd & Hermelin 1977). Deaf infants can become extremely sensitive to gesture, facial expression and the outcome of visual happenings (Schlesinger & Meadow 1972). The babble which deaf babies acquire was originally thought to disappear abruptly around 9 months of age (Lenneberg 1967) but recent research has noted the 'falling off' of the babble is more protracted than previously thought (Oller 1986). Mature babble of normal infants is multisyllabic with consonants and becomes ever more speech-like as the result of auditory feedback. Since auditory feedback is missing in the deaf baby, mature babble does not appear and their immature babble gradually fades away. This may be the ideal time for a deaf baby to learn sign language but depends upon an early diagnosis which is often extremely difficult to make. Parents of deaf babies talk to and imitate and repeat their baby's vocalizations less than the parents of hearing babies (Gregory et al 1979, 1981, Mogford 1988) presumably due to the lack of auditory feedback from their babies.

Expressive and receptive language development

Being without hearing does not preclude the development of language (Mogford 1988) but language will be delayed. Expressive, receptive and written language are all affected in deaf children. The speech production of deaf children affects vowels, consonants, tone, rhythm and voice quality. Intelligibility is a problem and semantics, rhyming (Dodd et al 1977) and syntax are all difficulties for deaf children. Deaf children make errors with verbs and tenses, leave off the ends of words, have a smaller vocabulary and performance does not improve with age (Nunnally & Blanten 1966). High-frequency deafness presents special problems. Only 47% of deaf 8-year-olds were intelligible to strangers (Martin & Moore 1979). The spoken language of deaf children shows delay rather than deviance and language development in the deaf is broadly similar to normal development except the acquisition of consonants is delayed (Abberton 1986). But even the understanding of vocabulary and underlying concepts is insufficient to help deaf children of good intelligence and moderate hearing losses with syntax (Quigley et al 1977). The level achieved is directly related to the degree of hearing loss. Deaf children use different strategies to normal children in written language whilst the understanding of grammar requires special tactics which the deaf may lack (Bishop 1983). Research into the reading and spelling of deaf children is sparse and the reason why some deaf children are good readers is not known (Freeman and Blockbuster 1987).

Inner or symbolic language

If not brain damaged, the deaf child can internalize visual and tactile sensations and integrate experientially, i.e behave symbolically. Hence their inner or symbolic language is good. Young deaf children play as imaginatively as hearing children (Newsom & Newsom 1979).

Motor function

The vestibular apparatus, in addition to the cerebellum, is involved in equilibrium so when vestibular function is disturbed, as it may be in some deaf children, motor function is inferior. Several studies have demonstrated

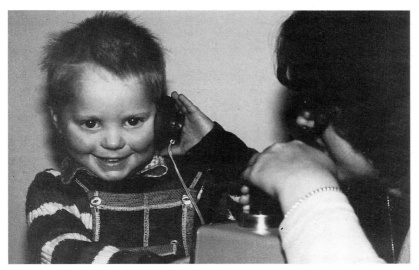

Fig. 11.12   'Playing' with Peter's mono-aural aged 25 months.

Assen's Play Audiometer

This audiometer is useful in the age range 3–7 years and has a range of 150–8000 Hz and 0–100 dB of pure tones and warbles. By pressing a knob when hearing the sound, a train and carriages are activated to travel round a circular track. The train *only* moves if a sound has been made so if restless children press the button indiscriminately the train does not move. Rather heavy headphones have to be accepted and train takes about 30 seconds to complete the circle and older children get bored after a few turns. Mentally retarded children frequently cannot be disciplined to press the button *only* when they hear a sound and misuse it. Sometimes they smile on hearing the sound, giving an indication that they heard it. This test is invaluable in language disordered and autistic children; indeed it might be argued that it is helpful in making a differential diagnosis as these children passively tolerate the headphones and respond by pressing the button correctly, seeming to enjoy the repetitious nature of the train movement and do not become bored. Several nonverbal children have been saved from a BSER because accurate audiograms have been obtained in this way.

Tympanometry

When a hearing loss is found it will be followed with tympanometry. Use of this technique in small babies has been questioned (McCormick 1986) but, if the baby is still and the mouth closed, a reading can be obtained in children of all ages. Results in babies under 3 months may be difficult to interpret, but a positive reading, especially a perfect acoustic reflex, which records the contraction of the stapedius muscle and implies integrity of the nerve pathway, is almost certainly correct. A positive result for the selected frequencies of the instrument can only be implied because there may be a recruitment problem. Children with a mental age of 18–24 months tolerate the procedure but children of 2+ years may require some guile to obtain compliance. Children coming for follow-up often enquire 'Are we going to play with your magic drawing machine?' Tympanometry gives useful information of middle ear function. A normal tympanogram and normal ear canal air pressure excludes a middle ear effusion (Fig. 11.13). A flat or 'type c' tympanogram with a mild-to-moderate hearing loss in the lower registers is confirmatory of a middle ear effusion (Fig. 11.14). Due to altered compliance of the eardrum, a poor acoustic reflex may also result but small waves are usually present in contradistinction to sensorineural deafness in which the reading is a completely straight line. If a middle ear effusion is improving the pressure curve is present but negative (Fig. 11.15) and may help to decide on a wait-and-see policy of treatment.

Speech and language tests

Comprehension, expression and symbolic language will be assessed (Ch. 9) but auditory discrimination and articulation tests are helpful in assessing hearing.

Auditory discrimination

The Goldman-Fristoe-Woodcock (1970) test of auditory discrimination consists of pages each of which has four acoustically similar pictures, e.g. pear; tear; hair; bear. A quiet voice pronounces one of the words and the child points to the appropriate picture. This procedure is

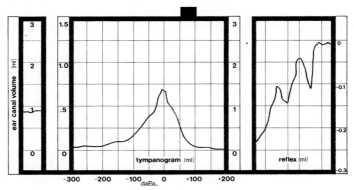

Fig. 11.13   Normal tympanogram.

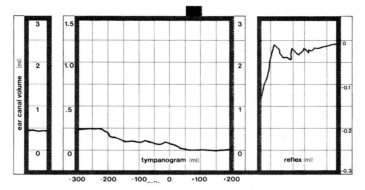

Fig. 11.14   Middle ear effusion tympanogram.

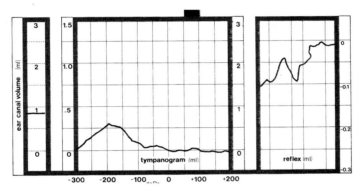

Fig. 11.15   Recovering 'glue' ear tympanogram.

repeated with the voice heard against a noisy background. The test distinguishes between poor auditory discrimination in a noisy environment and central discrimination, is age related and has percentile charts. For speech therapists or researchers, the sounds can be subdivided into speech types but for the DP it is a screening device. Finding a marked difference between the percentiles of the 'quiet' and 'noise' subtests suggests a conductive hearing loss whilst if both are poor, the diagnosis is more likely to be a central problem, i.e. language disorder or mental retardation.

The Toy discrimination test (McCormick 1977) is good for young children who have a mental age of 2yrs+ and mentally retarded children who will not undertake more complex tasks often cooperate. A sound meter is needed to monitor voice levels. There is no distinction between peripheral and central auditory reception and perception.

Articulation Tests

(See Ch. 9.) Children's articulatory defects are usually the result of poor auditory discrimination and a study of their mistakes can be revealing; e.g. 's', 'f', 't', short 'i' are characteristically high frequency sounds and deficient in this type of deafness; children with conductive losses will have problems with low frequency sounds, such as 'oo'. It will be remembered, however, that 's' and syllables with 's' and 'th' are the last to be learned and a lack may be within normal developmental level for young children.

IQ tests

Some IQ tests have been standardized for deaf and normally hearing children and the The Hiskey-Nebraska scale of learning *REF* is one such test.

DIFFERENTIAL DIAGNOSIS

Children with normal hearing may interpret sounds abnormally and children with mental retardation or behavioural problems may give inconsistent responses to sounds. Children with hearing losses cannot respond normally to sounds and may have abnormal hearing sensitivity.

Since the treatment and care of children with different problems differs, an accurate differential diagnosis is essential. The hearing loss in terms of pure tones has to be equated with ability to comprehend language and the child's own executive skills and this is only possible by assessing the whole child — his skills or deficits in all developmental parameters. The initial diagnosis is between a child who *cannot hear* or who *is not responding* to sounds. The latter is likely to be nonverbal or grossly language deficient. The differential diagnosis is therefore between deafness, language disorder/autism, mental retardation and, sometimes, behaviour problems. Table 11.5 is a resumé of the differential diagnosis with mild language delays not included because the differential diagnosis is not difficult. This differential diagnosis assumes that these four categories are 'pure', whilst in reality, this is frequently not the case, *viz*. the common association of deafness with mental retardation. All may have accompanying behaviour, social or familial problems. It is easier to exclude deafness as a diagnosis than to make the differential diagnosis.

TREATMENT, CARE AND EDUCATION

The aims of treatment are to:

- improve hearing
- develop communication, speech and language
- help the personality to grow

Table 11.5 Differential diagnosis between deafness, language disorder, mental retardation with no deafness, and behavioural disorder

	Deafness	Language disorder	Mental retardation with no deafness	Behaviour disorder
History	May be positive family history Maternal history drugs and/or infections	Usually unremarkable May be positive family history of late language development or learning problems	May be positive for: Inborn errors Genetic inheritance Consanguinity	History usually. non-contributory
Perinatal	Prematurity Kernicterus Apnoea Injury		Cerebral damage Hypoxia	May be low birthweight
Postnatal	Infections Drugs Trauma Late and abnormal language development	Late language development	Infections Trauma Severe deprivation	
Nonverbal skills	Normal	Average at first	Poor and delayed	Average if cooperation achieved
Hearing tests	*Mild conductive* Mild loss in lower frequencies Flat tympanogram Reduced ear canal air volume *High frequency loss* Moderate to severe loss in higher frequency Middle ear function normal *Sensorineural loss* Moderate to severe loss in many frequencies Absent tympanic reflex	Hearing normal May not respond to sounds Can be 'caught out' with unusual sounds Enjoy Assen's train audiometer Normal tympanogram, acoustic reflex May need AER to get evidence of normal hearing	Hearing normal May respond to test suitable for younger age group Cooperation may be difficult Satisfactory but responds as lower age group	Normal hearing Normal tympanogram May dislike loud noises

Table 11.5 (Contd).

	Deafness	Language disorder	Mental retardation with no deafness	Behaviour disorder
	Electrocochleography may show site of lesion AER slow wave V and SN10 no click intensity			
Auditory discrimination	Poor	Poor		
Gesture	Marked and good	Absent	No	Variable
Lipreading	Marked	Noticably absent Gaze avoidance	No	No Normal or gaze avoidance
Language	*Comprehension* Variable but below average *Expressive* Articulation, phonation and semantics poor *Symbolic*–excellent *Echolalia*–none	*Comprehension*–none or abnormal *Expression*–poor or none *Symbolic*–absent *Echolalia*–++++	*Comprehension*–poor *Expression*–poor but better than comprehension *Symbolic*–poor *Echolalia*–frequent	*Comprehension*–average *Expressive*–average *Symbolic*–average *Echolalia*–absent
Motor problems	Not marked but balance may be poor	Usually agile and graceful	May be best skill	Normal
Learning skills	*Reading* poor *Spelling* poor but better than reading *Mathematics* good	*Reading* may be fair but comprehension absent *Spelling* poor *Maths* poor	*Reading, spelling, maths* all below age	*Learning skills* unaffected or below average
Social behaviour	Aware of others May be reticent and shy Try to hear but cannot	Non-conversational Self-centred, no eye contact Socially insensitive Appear neither to hear nor listen May have inappropriate emotional response	Variable, may be friendly or inappropriate Hears but does not listen	Variable

Table 11.5 (*contd*).

	Deafness	Language disorder	Mental retardation with no deafness	Behaviour disorder
Attention	Excellent	May be unobtainable	Very poor. Distractible. Does not understand	Often distractible. Best in one-to-one situations
Reaction to environment	Unless recruitment problem, do not dislike noisy atmosphere or crowds	No eye contact but may look at inanimate objects	Often become confused and/or excited. Infantile hypocalcaemia, hypersensitive to home	Variable

- educate to potential
- assure a happy, well-adjusted person.

The treatment of hearing losses is the province of technical experts and cooperation with an audiologist, a peripetatic teacher of the deaf and sometimes an ENT surgeon is essential and their expertise invaluable. However, the aims stated above demonstrate the continued need for the involvement of a DP. Babies and children develop and their needs alter, their education needs planning and there is a constant need for reassessment if anything approaching the utopian ideals outlined are to be obtained. It has been stressed how important is an early diagnosis but there is an immediate divide amongst the experts as to which is the best treatment.

The oralist view (Freeman 1976) is that spoken language is all. It is argued that since most deaf children can be taught some language and to lip-read, the use of gesture and sign language only isolate the deaf from the hearing. This viewpoint sees amplification, lip-reading and auditory training as the bedrock of treatment and sign language and gesturing are frowned upon. There is disagreement which is the best time to start hearing aids and auditory training (Griffiths 1976) but the prevailing view is as early as possible (Drillien et al 1977). The oralists' view is a longer and, possibly, more uncertain route but the child is more likely to attend a normal school. The oralist view remains the consensus view in the UK (Ludman 1981). 53% of deaf children in the EEC countries were being educated by this method (Martin & Moore 1979). However, 64% of 8-year-olds had unintelligible speech, or speech which was defective and intelligible only to parents and, faced with a failure of their methods, oralists may have to resort to signing or manual methods of language.

The 'total communication' viewpoint helps the infant to acquire gesturing and sign language as soon as possible thus taking consideration of emotional and social needs. Since the early development of deaf babies with deaf mothers is better than that of deaf babies with hearing mothers it could be assumed that early gesturing and signing are helpful. Of course deaf mothers are more likely than hearing mothers to be proficient in these skills (Meadows 1969). A positive statement (e.g. Freeman & Blockberger 1987) that learning a sign language does not inhibit acquisition of speech and lip-reading has helped the oralists to accept this view. 'Total communicator' exponents see signing as a legitimate language. Some problems of signing languages are:

- parents have to learn to sign
- teachers have to be conversant with the method
- the child will probably be in a class with only other deaf children.

Following the diagnosis of deafness, procedure will be:

1. *Referral to otologist* (Ludman 1981). Seeking the cause and possible. treatment of the hearing condition is the realm of the otologist.

experiments on the development of language in deaf children. University of Illinois Institute of Research on Exceptional Children (Urbana champaign), Illinois

Breslaw P, Griffiths A, Wood D, Howarth C 1981 The referential communication skills of deaf children from different educational environments. Journal of Psychology and Psychiatry and Allied Disciplines 22: 269–282

Breslaw P I, Griffiths A J, Howarth C I 1981 The referential communication skills of deaf children from different environments. Journal of Child Psychology and Psychiatry and Allied Disciplines 22.3: 269–282

Brooks D N, Wooley H, Kanjilal G C 1972 Hearing loss and middle ear disorders in patients with Down's syndrome (mongolism). Journal of Mental Deficiency Research 16: 21–28

Campanelli P A, Pollock F J, Henner R 1958 An oto-audiological evaluation of 44 premature children. Archives of Otolaryngology 67: 609–615

Clements J 1987 Parental involvement in remediation for children with specific language disabilities. In: Proceedings of the First International Symposium on Specific Speech and Language Disorders in Children, Reading

Condon W S, Sander L W 1974 Neonate movement is synchronised with adult speech: interactional participation and language acquisition. Science 183: 99–101

Conrad R 1979 The deaf school child, Harper & Row, London

Cornforth A R T, Johnson K, Walker M 1974 The Makaton Vocabulary. Royal Association for Deaf People, London

Craig W N, Salem J M 1975 Partial integration of deaf with hearing students: residential school perspectives. American Annals of the Deaf 120: 28–36

Cunningham C, McArthur K 1981 Hearing loss and treatment in young Down's syndrome children. Child: Care, Health and Development 7: 357–374

Dale D M C 1978 Educating deaf and partially hearing children individually in ordinary schools. Lancet ii: 884–887

Darwin C 1965 The expression of the emotions in man and animals. University of Chicago Press, Chicago

Davies B 1988 Auditory disorders in Down's syndrome. Scandinavian Audiology suppl 30: 65–68

Dodd B, Hermelin B 1977 Phonological coding by the prelingually deaf. Perception and psychophysics 21: 413–417

Douck E, Bannister L H, Dodson H C, Ashcroft P, Humphries K N 1976 Effects of incubator noise on the cochlea of the newborn. Lancet ii: 1110–1113

Drillien C, Drummond M 1977 Hearing loss. In: Neurodevelopmental problems in early childhood: assessment and management. Blackwell Scientific Publication, Oxford

Eimas P D 1975 Speech perception in early infancy. In: Cohen L B, Salapatek P (eds) Perception. Academic Press, New York

Ewing A, Ewing E C 1971 Hearing impaired children under five. Manchester University Press, Washington

Fireman P 1988 Hayfever children get more earache. G P News, Oct 28

Fisher B 1966 The social and emotional adjustment of children with impaired hearing attending ordinary class. British Journal of Educational Psychology 36: 319–321

Fishman J E, Gadoth N, Radvan H 1983 Congenital sensorineural deafness associated with EEG abnormalities, epilepsy and high familial incidence. Developmental Medicine and Child Neurology 25: 747–754

Flood L M, Fraser J G, Conway M J, Stewart A 1982 The assessment of hearing in infancy using the Postauricular Myogenic Response. British Journal of Audiology 16: 211–214

Freeman R 1976 The deaf child: controversy over teaching methods. Journal of Child Psychology and Psychiatry and Allied Disciplines 17: 229–232

Freeman R, Blockberger S 1987 Language development and sensory disorder, visual and hearing impairments. In: Yule W, Rutter M (eds) Language development and disorders. MacKeith Press, Oxford

Freeman R D, Malkin S F, Hastings J O 1975 Psychosocial problems of deaf children and their families: comparative study. American Annals of the Deaf 121:391–405

Frostig M, Lefever W, Whittlesey J 1961 A developmental test of visual motor perception for evaluating normal and neurologically handicapped children. Perception and Motor Skills 12:52

Fry J, Dillane J B, Jones R F, McNab K, Kalton G, Andrew E 1969 The outcome of acute otitis media. British Journal of Preventive and Social Medicine 23: 205–209

Fry J 1987 The management of otitis media. Horizons: 163–170

Fulton R T, Lloyd L L 1968 Hearing impairment in a population of children with Down's syndrome. American Journal of Mental Deficiency 73: 298

Furth H G 1966 Thinking without language: psychological implications of deafness. Free Press, New York

Furth H G, Youniss J 1976 Formal operations: a comparison of deaf and hearing adolescents. In: Morehead M D, Morehead A (eds) Normal and deficient child language. University Park Press, Baltimore

Goetzinger C P 1962 Effects of small perceptive losses on language and on speech discrimination. Volta Review 64: 408–414

Goetzinger C P, Proud G O 1975 The impact of hearing impairment upon the psychological development of children. Journal of Auditory Research 15: 1–60

Goldman R, Fristoe M, Woodcock R W 1970 Test of auditory discrimination. American Guidance Service, Circle Pines, Minnesota

Graham N C 1970 The language of the educationally subnormal child. Final report to the Department of Education and Science, London

Gregory S 1976 The deaf child and his family. Wiley, Chichester

Gregory S, Mogford K 1981 Early language development in deaf children. In: Woll B, Kyle J, Deuchar M (eds) Perspectives on British sign language and deafness. Croom Helm, London

Gregory S, Mogford K, Bishop J 1979 Mothers' speech to young hearing impaired children. Journal of the British Association for Teachers of the Deaf 3: 42–43

Griffiths C 1975 The auditory approach: its rationale, techniques and results. Audiology and Hearing Education 1: 35–36, 38–39

Hall R, Richards H 1987 Hearing loss and mumps. Archives of Disease in Childhood 62: 189–203

Helms D B, Turner J S 1976 The sense of hearing: cognition and perception. In: Exploring child behaviour. W B Saunders, Philadelphia, p 117

Holm V A, Kunze H 1969 Effects of chronic otitis media on language and speech development. Pediatrics 45.5: 833–839

Holt K S 1977 Awareness: receiving and seeking sensory stimuli. Examination of receptive functions no 147. In: Holt K S (ed) Developmental paediatrics. Postgraduate Paediatrics Series. Butterworth, London

Hooker D 1952 The prenatal origin of behaviour. Lawrence/University of Kansas Press, Kansas

Horak F B, Shumway-Cook A, Crowe T K, Black F O 1988 Vestibular function and motor profiency of children with impaired hearing, or with learning disability and motor impairments. Developmental Medicine and Child Neurology 30: 64–79

Hosking C S, Pyman C, Wilkins B 1983 The nerve deaf child — intrauterine rubella or not? Archives of Disease in Childhood 58: 327–329

Howland A, Rasbury W, Heilman K M, Hammer L 1975 The development of auditory figure-ground discrimination and ear asymmetry under monoaural stimulus presentation. Developmental Medicine and Child Neurology 17: 325–332

Hyman C B, Keaster J, Hanson V, Harris I, Sedgwick R, Wursten H, Wright A N 1969 Abnormalities after neonatal hemolytic disease or hyperbilirubinemia. American Journal of Diseases of Children 117: 395–405

Ingram T T S 1959 Specific developmental disorders of speech in childhood. Brain 82: 450

Ives L A 1967 Deafness and the development of intelligence. British Journal of the Disorders of Communication 2: 2

Jaffe B F 1976 Pinna anomalies associated with congenital conductive hearing loss. Pediatrics 57: 332–341

Jones F E, Hanson D R 1977 *H. influenzae* meningitis treated with ampicillin or chloramphenicol and subsequent hearing loss. Developmental Medicine and Child Neurology 19: 593–597

Kaga R M, Suzuki J, Marsh R R, Tanaka Y 1981 Influence of labyrinthine hypoactivity on gross motor development of infants. Annals of New York Academy of Sciences 374: 412–420

Kahn A, Picard E, Blum D 1986 Auditory arousal thresholds of normal and near-miss SIDS infants. Developmental Medicine and Child Neurology 28: 299–302

Kantar R M, Clark D, Allen L C, Chase M F 1976 Effects of vestibular stimulation in nystagmus response and motor performance of developmentally delayed infants. Physical Therapy 59: 414–421

Keith R 1976 The use of impedance movements in infant hearing programs. In: Menche R G (ed) Early identification of hearing loss. Karger, Basel, pp 68–75

Keller W D, Bundy R S 1980 Effects of unilateral hearing loss upon educational achievement. Child: Care, Health and Development 6: 93–100

Kenyon G S 1988 Neuro-otological findings in normal children. Journal of the Royal Society of Medicine 81: 644–648

Kimura D 1964 Left–right differences in the perception of melodies. Quarterly Journal of Experimental Psychology 16: 355

Konigsmark B W, Gorlin R J 1976 Genetic and metabolic deafness. W B Saunders, Philadelphia

Lemon R E, Scott D M 1966 On the development of song in young cardinals. Canadian Journal of Zoology 44: 191–197

Lenneburg E H 1967 Biological foundations in the study of language. Wiley, New York

Lewis M M 1963 Language, thought and personality in infancy and childhood. Harrap, London

Lewis N 1976 Otitis media and linguistic incompetence. Archives of Otolaryngology 102: 387–390

Ludman H 1981 Deafness in childhood: ABC of ENT. British Medical Journal 282: 381–383

MacKeith R C, Rutter M 1972 A note on the prevalence of language disorders in young children. In: Rutter M, Martin J A M (eds) The child with delayed speech. Clinics in Developmental Medicine 43. Spastics International Medical Publications/Heinemann Medical Books, London

Marcus R E 1970 Reduced incidence of congenital and prelingual deafness. Archives of Otolaryngology 92: 343–347

Martin F N 1978 Etiology and pathology of hearing loss in children. In: Martin F N (ed) Pediatric audiology 4. Prentice Hall, Englewood Cliffs, New Jersey

Martin J A M 1977 Hearing loss. In: Drillien C M, Drummond M B (eds) Neurodevelopmental problems in early childhood. Blackwell Scientific Publications, Oxford

Martin J A M, Moore W J 1979 Childhood deafness in the European Community. Commission of the European Communities (EUR 6413)

Mason S, McCormick B, Wood S 1988 Auditory brainstem response in paediatric audiology. Archives of Disease in Childhood 63: 465–460

McAndrew H 1948 Rigidity in the deaf and blind. Journal of Social Issues 4: 72

McCormick B 1977 The Toy Discrimination Test — an aid for screening the hearing of children above a mental age of 2 years. Public Health London 91: 73–76

McCormick B 1986 Hearing screening for the very young. In: Meadow R (ed) Recent advances in paediatrics. Churchill Livingstone, Edinburgh

McCormick B, Curnock D A, Spavins F 1984 Auditory screening of special care neonates using the auditory response cradle. Archives of Disease in Childhood 59: 1168–1172

McDonald A D 1989 Deafness in children of very low birth weight. Archives of Disease in Childhood 64: 1646

McFie J 1973 Musical behaviour in early childhood. Developmental Medicine and Child Neurology 15: 848–849

Meadow S K 1968 Toward a developmental understanding of deafness. Journal of Rehabilitation of the Deaf 2: 1

Ministry of Education 1963 Report on a survey of deaf children who have been transferred from special schools or units to ordinary schools. HMSO, London

Ministry of Education 1964 Survey of children born in 1947 who were in schools for the deaf in 1962–3. In: The health of the school child: report of the Chief Medical Officer of the Dept of Education and Science for the years 1962 and 1963. HMSO, London

Miyawaki K, Strange W, Verbrugge R, Liberman A M, Jenkins J J, Fujimura D 1975 An effect of linguistic experience: the discrimination of 'r' and 'l' by native speakers of Japanese and English. Perception and Psychophysics 18: 331–340

Mogford K 1988 Oral language acquisition in the prelinguistically deaf. In: Bishop D, Mogford K (eds) Language development in exceptional circumstances. Churchill Livingstone, Edinburgh

Morris D 1978 Manwatching: A field guide to human behaviour. Triad Panther, St Albans

Morsch J 1936 Motor performance of the deaf. Comparative Psychology Monographs 66:

Mozart W A 1789 K 581 Quintet for Clarinet and Strings in A flat

Myklebust H R 1954 Auditory disorders in children. Grune & Stratton, New York

Myklebust H R 1964 Significance of etiology in motor performance of deaf children with special reference to meningitis. American Journal of Psychology 59: 249

Newsom E, Newsom J 1979 Using toys and play remedially. In: Newsom J, Newsom E (eds) Toys and playthings in development and remediation. Allen & Unwin, London

Newton V 1985 Aetiology of bilateral sensorineural hearing loss in young children. Journal of Laryngology and Otology, suppl 10

Nietupska O, Harding N 1982 Auditory screening of school children: fact or fallacy? British Medical Journal 284: 717–720

Northcott W H 1973 The hearing impaired child in a regular classroom. A G Bell Association for the Deaf, Washington DC

Northern J, Downs M 1974 Hearing in children. Williams & Wilkins, Baltimore

Nottebohm F, Nottebohm M E 1971 Vocalizations and breeding behaviour of surgically deafened ring doves. Animal Behaviour 19: 313–327

Nunnally J C, Blanton R L 1966 Patterns of word association in the deaf. Psychological Reports 18: 87–92

O'Connor N, Hermelin B 1978 Seeing and hearing and space and time. Academic Press, London, pp 307–318

Oller D K 1986 Metaphonology and infant vocalisation. In: Lindblom B, Zetterstrom R (eds) Precursors of early speech. Macmillan, Basingstoke

Paget R, Gorman P, Paget G 1976 The Paget Gorman Sign System. Association for Experiment in Deaf Education, London

Paradise J L 1981 Otitis media during early life. How hazardous to development? A critical review of the evidence. Pediatrics 68: 869–873

Peckham C S, Sheridan M D 1976 Follow-up at 11 years of 46 children with severe unilateral hearing loss at 7 years. Child: Care, Health and Development. 2: 107–111

Pintner R, Lev J 1939 The intelligence of the hard of hearing school child. Journal of Genetic Psychology 55: 31–48

Pollak M, Thomas N 1993 Glue ears, grommets and language development (in press)

Prior M R, Glazner J, Sanson A, Debelle G 1988 Research note. Temperament and behavioural adjustment in hearing impaired children. Journal of Child Psychology and Psychiatry and Allied Disciplines 29.2: 209–216

Quigley S P, Power D J, Steinkamp M W (1977) The language structure of deaf children. Volta Review 79: 73–84

Quigley S T 1978 Effects of early hearing on normal language development. In: Martin F N (ed) Pediatric audiology. Prentice Hall Englewood Cliffs, New Jersey

Rapin I 1979 Conductive hearing loss effects on children's language and scholastic skills: a review of the literature. Annals of Otology, Rhinology and Laryngology 88 Suppl 60 P 2

Rubein R J, Rapin I 1980 Plasticity of the developing auditory system. Annals of Otology 89: 303–311

Rutter M 1972 The effects of language delay on development. In: Rutter M, Martin J A M (eds) The child with delayed speech. Clinics in Developmental Medicine 43. Spastics International Medical Publications/Heinemann Medical Books, London

Scanlon P E, Bamford J M 1990 Early identification of hearing loss: screening and surveillance methods. Archives of Disease in Childhood 65.5: 479–486

Schein F N, Delk M T 1974 The deaf population of the United States. Silver Spring Medical National Association of the Deaf

Schlesinger H S, Meadow K P 1972 Sound and sign: childhood deafness and mental health. University of California, Berkeley

Sheridan M D 1964 Development of auditory attention and language symbols in young children. In: Renfrew C, Murphy K (eds) The child who does not talk. Clinics in Developmental Medicine. Spastics International Medical Publications/Heinemann Medical Books, London, p 3

Sheridan M D 1972 Reported incidence of hearing loss in children of 7 years. Developmental Medicine and Child Neurology 14: 296–303

Strange W, Jenkins J J 1978 Role of linguistic experience in the perception of speech. In: Walk R D, Pick H L (eds) Perception and experience. Plenum, New York

Thiringer K, Kankunen A, Niklasson A 1984 Perinatal risk factors in the aetiology of hearing loss in preschool children. Developmental Medicine and Child Neurology 26: 799–807

Turkewitz G, Birch H G, Cooper K K 1972 Patterns of response to different auditory stimuli in the human newborn. Developmental Medicine and Child Neurology 14: 487–491

van Uden A M J 1983 Diagnostic testing of deaf children — the syndrome of dyspraxia. Lisse, Swets & Zeitlinger

van Zyl F J, Ives L A 1971 Visual perception and eye-motor co-ordination in a group of young deaf children. Developmental Medicine and Child Neurology 13: 373–379

Vanderschueren-Lodeweyckx M, Debruyne F, Dooms L, Eggermont E, Eeckels R 1983 Sensorineural hearing loss in sporadic congenital hypothyroidism. Archives of Disease in Childhood 58: 419–422

Vuori M, Lahikainen E A, Pettonen T 1962 Perceptive deafness in connection with mumps. Acta Otolaryngologica 55: 231–236

Walk R D 1981 Perceptual development. Brook/Cole, Monterey, California

Weston P, Weinman J 1983 The effects of auditory and linguistic deprivation on lateral preference of deaf children. Developmental Medicine and Child Neurology 25: 207–213

Wiegersma P H, van Der Velde A 1983 Motor development of deaf children. Journal of Child Psychology and Psychiatry and Allied Disciplines 24.1: 103–111

Wild N J, Sheppard S, Smithells R W, Holzel H, Jones G 1989 Onset and severity of hearing loss due to congenital rubella infection. Archives of Disease in Childhood 64: 1280–1283

Wood D J, Wood H A, Griffiths A J, Howarth S P, Howarth C I 1982 The structure of conversations with 6–10 year old deaf children. Journal of Child Psychology and Psychiatry and Allied Disciplines 23: 295–308

Yeates S 1980 Development of hearing. In: Pollak M (ed) Studies in developmental paediatrics, vol 2. MTP Press, Lancaster

Yule W, Udwin O 1987 The role and value of augmented communication. In: Proceedings of the First International Symposium on Specific Speech and Language Disorders in Children. HGA Printing Co, Brentford for AFASIC, London

Zielhuis G A, Rach G H, van den Broek P 1989 Screening for otitis media with effusion in preschool. Lancet i: 311–313

Zincus P W, Gottlieb M I, Schapiro M 1978 Developmental and psychoeducational sequelae of chronic otitis media. American Journal of Diseases of Children 321: 1100–1104

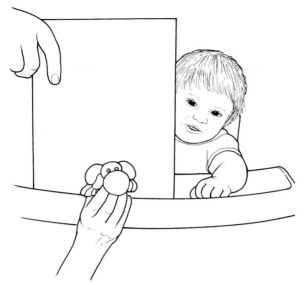

Fig. 12.5   Pushing the screen aside—understands object permanence, over 4 months old.

struggled to test far vision will know only too well, it is difficult to sustain this interest for much longer than a minute at 3 or 6 metres distance. Eye-motor coordination is now such that he automatically reaches out to the objects and displays his new-found skill of pointing with index finger. He looks to see where dropped toys and objects have fallen. Indeed, his favourite game is casting toys out of pram or cot so that someone will pick them up and replace them and he can repeat the performance! He easily distinguishes between mother, father, siblings and strangers. There is a colour preference for red and yellow — a fact of which designers of nurseries and children's toys and clothes seem unaware. Pastels are for fairy tales.

Over 1 year: At 1 year the pupils have enlarged and central acuity is 20/100. It is only after 1 year that the concept of two dimensions is fully understood. Although depth perception has been present for some time, he still may look behind the television to see the back of the person on the screen and, before this skill is acquired, he tries to 'pick out' a person or animal from a picture book.

Visual acuity

Opinion is divided on the time at which full adult visual acuity is acquired. Sheridan (1974) asked several ophthalmologists what they considered normal visual acuity at 5 years of age. The estimates varied from 6/9 to 6/18 and such views can still be read in textbooks of ophthalmology. Sheridan (1973) tested 100 schoolchildren aged 5–7 years. 83% had a visual acuity of 6/4.5. In her opinion, (Sheridan 1974) at age 5, 6/9 in both eyes requires follow-up and 6/12 in one eye referral. Moreover, she believed that 6/9–6/9 at this age represents functional immaturity rather than structural defect and might, therefore, be indicative of early myopia. Ikeda (1979) estimated that visual acuity in man should be complete by 2 years. Catford & Oliver (1973) and Holt (1975) tacitly agree and estimated human visual acuity as follows:

- at 5 months: 6/18
- at 18 months: 6/9
- at 3 years: 6/6.

Using visual evoked response techniques on babies aged 1 to 7 months of age, visual acuity was 20/400 at 1 month and adult (20/20) at 6 months (Marg et al 1976). Sheridan (1973) was convinced that 6/6 is normal towards the end of the second year of life and this author is in agreement. It may well be earlier. These differences of opinion are important, however, because they affect clinical judgement of what is abnormal at a given age and, even more importantly, whether or not correction is required. Although the neonate's eye is hypermetropic, his rapidly developing powers of accommodation overcome this by appropriately refracting light to fall on the retina. When he becomes emmetropic accommodation is not required. But if the eye is myopic, accommodation will not help and blurred vision results. Improved vision includes the ability to discriminate very fine detail with increasing accuracy and speed. By 5–6 years of age children can discriminate forms from a background, i.e. figure-ground discrimination. Eye-sighting preference certainly occurs by age 5 years if not before. Thus, children from a young age possess adult vision; what matures is the ability to distinguish the finer detail of visual perception.

FACTORS AFFECTING DEVELOPMENT OF NORMAL VISION

Maturity

Under 31 weeks gestational age, the discriminative visual function of tracking or visual preference is not present nor are babies able to focus (Dubowitz et al 1980).

Development

Visual acuity develops as a result of the use of vision, sharp retinal images being due to development of the macula and the ability of the lens to accommodate. The development of visual acuity therefore depends upon the accurate and normal development of these structures. A child with a high refractive error will not receive sharp retinal images and this lack of 'practice' produces a functional amblyopia which requires early correction in order that the retina can receive sharp images. Late treatment of congenital cataracts, for example, results in low visual acuity for this reason. Alternating esotropia is the rule which, if monocular, results in the eye not being used which causes arrested visual development.

Interaction with other humans

A baby needs to have someone (probably his mother) to visually focus on the same object as that at which he is looking, a phenomenon known as visual coorientation. The mother then looks at her baby who responds by looking back at her. Social interaction begins and is enhanced. These visual responses of a baby and his mother are not, as might be supposed, independent of each other (Collis & Schaffer 1975)and babies who do not experience this personal visual interplay, e.g. those brought up in institutions, are less visually curious and responsive and seek visual eye-catching to a lesser degree than babies who experience it frequently.

Movement

Movement is important since visual interest is aroused by moving contours in the visual field, a fact made use of in optokinetic nystagmus. Movement is particularly important in the development of visual perception as animal experiments suggest. Cats, for example, who can see but not move do not develop depth perception and it has been hypothesized this might also apply to humans (Held & Hein 1963). However, whilst agreeing that movement is essential for depth perception, Walk (1981) argues the baby does not need to move; exposure to a movement in the visual field has the same effect. He cites paralysed but well-stimulated babies who develop perception of depth. Thalidomide children who, although born without arms and legs, nevertheless develop depth perception (Gouin-Decarie 1969) support this view.

Delayed dendritic and synaptic formation in visual cortex

This is thought to be a reason for delayed visual maturation (Cole et al 1984).

Drugs in labour

Some anaesthetic drugs given during labour alter the neonate's pattern preferences but the effect is short-lived (Blair et al 1984).

Experience

That the natural terrain of a child's environment may affect his ability to recognize horizontal and vertical orientation compared with the oblique is an interesting suggestion. It is argued that the predominating orientation of city life is the horizontal and vertical whilst this is not the case in a more natural terrain. Cree Indians, compared to children living in highrise flats in a city, are highly superior in detecting oblique structures and it has been postulated that a 'carpentered' environment, i.e. one full of horizontal and vertical lines (Fig. 12.6). makes city children susceptible to these lines whilst the Indians, living in wigwams, are more used to and therefore recognize more the oblique (Annis & Frost 1972). Perhaps a somewhat far-fetched theory but it receives support from the study of Timney & Muir (1976) who found that Chinese, who are good at recognizing obliques, lost this ability when they went to live in high-rise dwellings in Hong Kong.

ABNORMAL VISION

A child's vision is subjected to many conditions and abnormalities and if one considers the delicate balance between growth and accommodation

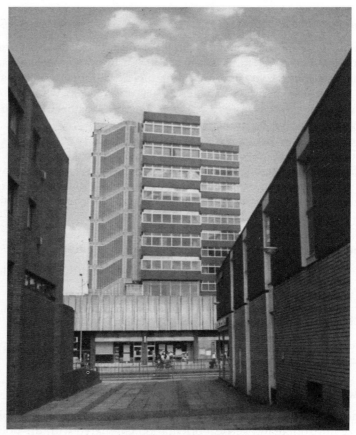

Fig. 12.6   The vertical and horizontal line of a city.

which occurs during development, the wonder is that any child has normal vision. It is neither possible nor appropriate to include all these conditions and the following are some of the more common and/or important visual defects of childhood.

Slow visual awareness

Some babies seem slow to become visually aware and Illingworth (1961) coined the phrase 'delayed visual maturation' for such babies, the inference being that, although they appear blind neonatally, they eventually develop vision. If they are of normal intelligence vision occurs around 6 months and later if developmentally delayed. However, at later follow-up, a high proportion have language or general developmental delay (Fielder et al 1985) and three have been described who became autistic (Goodman & Ashby 1990).

Refractive errors

Refractive errors are the most common visual problem of childhood. Refraction is the power of a transparent object to bend light rays. In the eye, this depends upon the curvature of surfaces and their distance from each other. Measurement of refraction includes these factors (Fig. 12.7). The antero-posterior axis determines whether the eye is hypermetropic, emmetropic or myopic. If the eye is healthy the refractive error can be corrected by wearing lenses. Hypermetropia with which babies are born slightly increases up to the age of 3, thereafter decreasing. 75% of 1000 neonates were hypermetropic and 25% myopic (Cook & Glassock 1951). The hypermetropia is compensated by accommodation and does not need correction but the 25% who are myopic require careful follow-up as the myopia will increase with age, may lead to retinal detachment or amblyopia and spectacles will be required.

Astigmatism

Astigmatism is a refractive error in which the difference between the vertical and horizontal meridians is markedly different causing inaccurate focusing which can be corrected by glasses. Refractive errors are associated with IQ and educational attainment. In the NCDS, 11-year-old myopes had higher reading ages; were better at maths and had general higher educational attainment than children who were not myopic (Peckham et al 1977) — a finding confirmed by Stewart-Brown et al (1985) and pre-myopic children have the edge on children who do not become myopic (Karlsson 1975). Children who were hypermetropic had lower verbal and performance scores than children with no refractive errors (Williams et al 1988). Myopia has also been associated with social

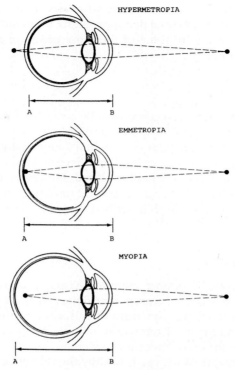

Fig. 12.7 Hypermetropia, emmetropia and myopia (From Gardiner PA 1982 Development and Vision. Studies in Developmental Paediatrics 3, MTP Press, Lancaster, courtesy of Kluwer Academic Publishers).

class. At age 11, NCDS children with myopia were more likely than those with no refractive error to have a father in a non-manual occupation (Peckham et al 1977).

Squints

Strabismus is an abnormal alignment of the eyes which prevents single binocular vision. Central fixation begins by 3–4 months and accurate alignment is needed for single binocular vision. Squint is due to incorrect binocular fixation with a resultant lack of stereoptic vision. This fixation reflex may be due to an abnormality of the sensory, motor or central coordinating part of the reflex. *Sensory* abnormalities are the more important for future outlook and are due either to high refractive errors or poor transparency of the media. Squints may result from corneal opacities, congenital vitreous defects, cataracts, diseases of the retina, tumours and optic atrophy. *Motor* abnormalities are conditions which interfere with extraocular muscle coordination such as 3rd, 4th and 6th cranial nerve defects. The strabismus may be concomitant or incomitant. The former is usually due to a refractive error or, unusually, to a neurological deficit due to a nerve palsy or pathology of the globe. It is necessary in a case of strabismus to ensure there is no underlying pathology and the strabismus is corrected at an early age to prevent amblyopia. Refraction and/or retinoscopy is a sine qua non. 3% of children have some type of strabismus and there is a strong familial tendency. 20.9% of 7-year-olds who had or had ever had a squint, had a difference of more than one line on visual testing compared with 2.3% who had never had a squint (Alberman et al 1971).

Nystagmus

Eye movements can be divided into those of:

1. *Fixation* which are high frequency, to and fro movements of small amplitude and keep the eye in the direction of the object on which fixation is required.
2. *Congugation* which bring the eye into a new direction, e.g. Cogan's ocular motor apraxia (see below).
3. *Dysjunction* which change the degree of convergence.

Nystagmus is a rhythmic to and fro oscillation of the eyes which may be *pendular* with movements of equal amplitude and rate or *jerky* with a rapid movement in one direction and a slower one in the other. The latter tends to occur in cerebellar or labyrinthine disease. Nystagmus is frequently secondary to *visual impairment* especially when the visual loss occurs congenitally or is acquired during the first year of life. Nystagmus may be associated with blindness, congenital cataracts, bilateral toxoplasmosis retinitis and severe rubella embryopathy. When visual loss affects the fovea rather than the peripheral retina and the pathology affects the anterior rather than posterior visual pathways, the resultant nystagmus is conjugate, being equal in frequency and amplitude. Roving eye movements may also be seen. If vision improves, the nystagmus becomes more rapid and smaller in amplitude. Convergence helps to suppress nystagmus. The quality of the nystasgmus is determined by the better eye, a fact which has been used to identify which eye has the better foveal vision (Jan et al 1988).

A *congenital* form of nystagmus, seen during the first month of life, is associated with hyper photosensitivity and is seen in ocular albinism or achromatopsia. Children often adopt head postures and tilting. A condition with characteristic random eye movements and voluntary vertical gaze has been described which is more common in males and shows some improvement with age (Cogan 1952). It is considered to be a congenital condition (Jan 1990) and an occurrence in two generations of a consanguinous family has been described (Vassella et al 1972). *Latent* nystagmus is congenital in origin and usually associated with esotropia. Seen when one eye is covered, the uncovered eye develops a jerky nystagmus which disappears when the cover is removed.

Acquired nystagmus may be unilateral and is seen either with associative neurological disease or following severe visual loss. When present from birth it is probably hereditary but acquired nystagmus is likely to be due to poor visual sensory input — a deprivation amblyopia. Lack of stimulation, from whatever cause, leads to abnormalities of the afferent visual pathways and visual cortex. Children with sensory and motor nystagmus sometimes show head shaking which is believed to be under voluntary control and is an attempt to improve visual fixation and vision. There is accompanying head tilting (Jan et al 1990).

Amblyopia

Amblyopia is usually defined as a reduction of 2+ lines on the Snellen's visual acuity chart. Traditionally subdivided into organic and inorganic, the latter is the more common. The visual loss can vary from minimal to blindness. *Inorganic* loss is usually a functional amblyopia caused by a squint or by the reflex of fusion not developing. *Uniocular* diminution of vision does not allow 'practice' and normal vision does not develop. Stimulation of the poorer eye is the basis of patching the better eye in strabismus.

Blindness

The definition of blindness is a matter of dispute — with 65 different definitions throughout the world (Freeman 1978). Most 'blind' persons have some residual vision and are, in fact, 'partially sighted'. An extremely sensible definition based on practical outcome is: those with visually directed reach and those dependent upon tactile location (Zinkin 1979). Blindness is *central* or *peripheral* in type.

Central blindness affects the perception of light, direction, shape, brightness, colour and movement. It is variable so children may see one thing and not another or can see one moment and not another. Since the lesion is sited at or between the geniculate bodies and the occipital cortex, pupils are intact and there is no optic atrophy. Damage is usually extensive and children are frequently mentally retarded. They rarely have roving movements and do not 'look blind' but appear inattentive and listless. Central blindess is *congenital* or *acquired* and may be *transient* or *permanent*. Central blindness is occasionally due to delayed developmental maturation and a neonate who appears blind may afterwards develop normal vision (Illingworth 1961) — see note above. *Congenital* central blindness is due to malformations or intrauterine infections which are the more

In the UK in 1968, 0.34 per 100 000 children aged 0–14 years were registered as blind and suffering from optic atrophy (Taylor 1975). The prevalence of severe visual disability in the preschool years is 1 in 3000 approximately (Sorsby 1972). Figure 12.8 shows the blind registrations of children 1948–1968, the increase in retrolental fibroplasia being the reason for the peak in 1953. The gradual overall decrease is due to the use of antibiotics and attention paid to oxygen levels during parturition. Congenital prenatal abnormalities account for the highest majority of blindness in children — 70% in this study.

In Holland, Lower-Sieger (1975), reporting on partially sighted or blind children aged 6–18 years attending special schools, found 63% were mentally normal and 37% mentally retarded. Children with congenital cataracts were those most likely to have normal intelligence. A breakdown of the causes was as follows:

- 19% were *tapetoretinal dystrophies* (this term describes hereditary degenerative conditions which affect the retina and, occasionally, the choroid. Tapetum refers to the tapetum nigrum pigment of epithelium of the retina. It is now known that retinal degeneration is not confined to this layer)
- 17% had *congenital cataracts*, 33% of which were transmitted by a defective gene
- 16% suffered *optic nerve atrophy*
- 15% had *malformations*
- 8% had *retrolental fibroplasia*
- 6% *albinism*.

A large number of the children had additional handicaps: 22% having important somatic defects; 18% motor deficits and 4% hearing losses. The aetiology of the severe visual impairments was striking, 91% of the total school population had a pre- or perinatal cause of which 49% were genetic in origin.

In Sweden the incidence of visual handicap in children aged 10–14 years is 1 per 1000 and 0.1 per 1000 for total blindness (Lindstedt 1975). 75% of children with residual vision have sufficient to allow perception of figures. Affections of the *retina and optic nerve* were the cause of most blindness with cataract and high refractive errors the least. Aetiology of the handicap was most often prenatal and manifest at birth. High refractive errors, either as a single cause or as an additional symptom, were present in 30% of visually handicapped children.

The prevalence of colour blindness

6% of boys and 1% of girls aged 11 year had a red/green problem (Peckham et al 1975).

CONDITIONS ASSOCIATED WITH VISUAL PROBLEMS

Cerebral palsy

Strabismus is the most common visual abnormality of cerebral palsy occurring in 40–60% of children (Duckman 1979). A dyskinetic strabismus is occasionally the first sign of cerebral palsy. Strabismus may account for the frequent learning problems which cerebral palsied children experience (Ayres 1972, Katayama & Tamas 1987). Diplegics and quadriplegics are particularly liable to visual abnormalities due to the tendency of the lesions to concentrate in the posterior parts of the hemispheres (Taudorf 1984). Visual acuity may be normal but difficulty in tracking and placing occur (Damasio & Benton 1979). Some cerebral palsied children suffer from visual inattention with resultant inability to aim and move the eyes where they want. Visuospatial difficulties (Rondot et al 1977) and refractive errors are common. Uncorrected strabismus may result in amblyopia.

Brain damage

Brain damage resulting from anoxia from any cause is commonly associated with complex visual disorders. The area of damage affects the type of lesion suffered and the injury itself delays myelinization (Dubowitz & Bydder 1985). With increasing ability to diagnose the site of the injury, prediction of the type of visual damage becomes increasingly accurate and depends whether it involves the *first visual system* — the optic radiation and area striata — or the *second visual system* — the parietal border zones. The former is responsible for precise identification of objects via macular and peripheral vision, whilst the latter (colliculo-pulvinar parietal projection) is responsible for direction of gaze and identification of objects which movements bring into view (Foley 1987).

Oxygen

The part played by oxygen in visual retinopathy is slightly more controversial than previously thought. Retrolental fibroplasia was thought to be entirely preventable (Kinsey 1956) provided premature babies were not exposed to high concentrations of oxygen and, following the restriction of oxygen, the incidence fell during the 1940s and '50s. However, there has been a rise in the '70s and '80s and cases occur when no excess oxygen has been given. New techniques, which allow study of the immature fundus, demonstrate that the blood supply of the preterm retina comes from choroidal vessels which are unable to constrict. Vasoconstriction of the retina may be a normal physiological reaction to protect the retina from hyperoxia and the premature retina cannot react in this way (Silverman 1982). Fielder et al (1986) suggest that it is developmental age

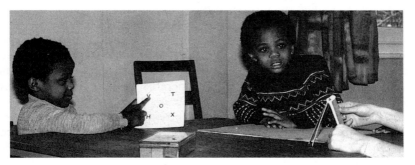

Fig. 12.13   3-year-old with Stycar five-letter test.

When the key card is replaced by plastic letters the majority of *30-month-old* children match by holding up or pointing to the plastic letter which matches the examiner's (Egan & Brown 1984). A recent updating of the Stycar tests which retains the developmental features but lessens the complexity is the *Sonksen-Silver acuity system* (Sonksen & Macrae 1987).

Tests of colour vision are of two types: those which arrange different hues in chromatic order and those which depend upon recognition of a different but allied colour from a coloured background. The latter are known as 'confusion' tests of which the *Isihara* test is the best known but expensive and time-consuming. The quicker and cheaper *Sheridan-Gardiner test of colour vision* is more widely used (Gardiner 1973). Children under 4 years of age dislike both tests.

Test for eye preference. The test is usually for a positive finding and performed by noting which eye is used for unilateral looking, e.g. a kaleidoscope. Peters (1975) found an association between crossed laterality and learning disabilities and incomplete dominance of one hemisphere was considered to account for some learning difficulties. However this finding has not been reproduced and an absence of eye preference or the presence of crossed laterality is probably of no significance. Hemiplegic children usually have an eye preference on the side of their lesion suggesting it is unrelated to one-sided hemispheric dominance (Costeff et al 1988).

Stycar panda test (Sheridan 1973). Designed for children with severe visual handicaps, this is similar to the Stycar letter tests but relies upon white letters and lines on a black ground, the very large letters are equivalent to 6/60. This test is useful for children who may have been labelled 'untestable'.

Reynell–Zinkin developmental scales (Reynell et al 1975). Theoretically of great help to developmentalists since the motor and mental development of the visually handicapped child is measured but they are incomplete and the equipment has to be individually assembled.

Preferential looking tests. When shown a bold and plain pattern a baby prefers to look at the former. If the bold pattern is a grating on which the lines become increasingly smaller, they eventually approach the 'dullness' of the latter. By noting the stage at which a baby becomes disinterested, it has been possible to standardize the grating to give a measure of visual acuity. The apparatus needs a special room, is immobile and expensive but has been used with considerable success (e.g. Dobson & Teller 1978, Mayer & Dobson 1982, Teller et al 1986).

Acuity cards. These cards are an alternative to preferential looking tests which are expensive, bulky and non-portable. They consist of grey cardboard in which there are two circular holes and a central peephole. The child sits facing the card at a defined distance. One of the holes has an extremely fine and unresolvable grating and the other shows vertical black and white waves of varying widths. The examiner watches the child's eyes through the central peephole. These cards have been used with a variety of children, e.g. neonates (Dobson et al 1987); children with Down syndrome (Hertz 1987); cerebral visual impairment (Hertz 1988); nonverbal children (Mohn 1988) and cerebral palsy and mentally retarded children of different aetiologies (Hertz 1988). They need to be more widely available (Teller et al 1986).

Videorefraction (Atkinson et al 1984). This is a new and hopeful method of testing infants and young children by the technique of photo-refraction. Accommodation as well as static refraction can be tested. Research suggests that babies under one year of age who show extreme hypermetropia are 20 times more likely to develop strabismus or amblyopia than emmetropic babies. It is quick and, with a built-in computer, gives an instant result. It is no doubt the technique of the future.

Electroretinogram (ERG) assesses the function of rods and cones by light stimulation in the retina. The ERG response is extinguished early in generalized tapetoretinal degeneration and the electroretinogram is altered by opacities and may be abnormal in congenital amaurosis before routine ophthalmic examination shows abnormality. It is considered of special use in children (Wybar & Harcourt 1970, Galloway 1979).

Visually evoked response (VER) is a cortical potential from an intermittent light stimulus. Electrodes are fitted on the scalp around the occipital lobe and patients exposed to flashes of light. The electrical responses are subsequently averaged out by computers. VER can be used to measure infant acuity but its most frequent use is for the diagnosis of cortical blindness. It has been used for the diagnosis of Tay-Sachs disease (Honda & Sudo 1976); to predict recovery (Tepperberg et al 1977) and for evaluating sensorimotor pathways in the neonate's brain (Klimach & Cooke 1988).

Babies who show no visual interest during the first 3 months of life have been described. Mellor & Fielder (1980) describe the follow-up of four such babies and, initially, all had unequivocally normal ERGs but absent, impaired or immature VERs. A gradual improvement over the next 12 weeks ensued and eventually all were visually (and generally) normal. The advantage of use of both methods of examination in doubtful cases is thus illustrated.

Computerized axial tomography (CAT) can be used to demonstrate the site and extent of a lesion (Tepperberg et al 1977) and occipital atrophy.

Angiography can be useful in cases of central cortical blindness where collections of pus or perfusion of the peripheral cortex may be demonstrated.

Visual evoked potential mapping and CT. A more recent technique, this has shown that children's cortical blindness has several subgroups not previously suspected (Whiting et al 1985).

Adaptations of existing tests. There has been the custom in tests to omit any visual component in IQ tests in children with visual problems. Groenveld (1990) is rightly critical of this practice as it assumes the experience, except for lack of vision, of a visually impaired child is the same as a normally sighted child. There are adaptations of existing IQ tests for the visually handicapped, e.g. the *Interim Hayes Binet test (IHB)* is an adaptation of the Binet-Simon with visual tests replaced by verbal material. There are problems with adaptations, e.g. the verbal skills of children need to be good; some of the tests are boring and most do not measure motor development. *Newlands blind learning aptitude test (BLAT)* correlates well with Binet and Wechsler tests (Dauterman et al 1967). There are three-dimensional adaptations of the *Raven's Progressive Matrices* and *Kohs Block Design test*. An adaptation of the *Vineland Social Maturity scales* may show if a child is lacking in initiative and independence. The *Williams test* (1957) has been devised for partially sighted or blind children and adapted from the Terman-Merrill test but tests are not scored. A study of subtest results may indicate which is the area of greatest problem (Bateman 1965). For a good description of psychological tests for visually impaired children see Tillman (1967a, b). The problem of these tests is the assumption that all handicapped children are the same and of normal intelligence.

Sonksen's Picture Test. Preschool children with refractive errors have a difficulty in seeing pictures and the use of pictures of increasing complexity may form the basis of a test for younger children (Sonksen et al 1987).

Effects of visual abnormalities

The effects of suboptimal visual acuity vary with severity and type of problem.

14% of normal schoolchildren in the NCDS had less than optimal vision but only those with hypermetropia were underachieving in reading. The mothers of children with visual defects considered them less able at sports than their visually perfect peers and to gain from wearing their prescribed spectacles (Stewart-Brown et al 1985). Children in the same study with *strabismus* were educationally disadvantaged (Alberman et al 1971).

IQ

Myopia and pre-myopia are associated with higher verbal, performance, reading and arithmetic scores at age 11 (Peckham et al 1977) and 17–18 years (Karlsson 1975) whilst *hypermetropia* is associated with slightly lower scores (Williams et al 1988). There may be a synergistic effect in mentally handicapped children with a visual problem whose visual acuity and developmental levels are lower than in a child with a deficiency in each separately (Warburg 1975) but this might be the result of not using developmentally based scales (Ellis 1978).

Blindness

The effect on development of being blind since birth is a matter of dispute. Some claim that blind children have no more psychological problems than the sighted (Schnittjer & Hirshoren 1981); others that blindness is an irreparable disaster (Fraiberg 1977), whilst others take a middle view that, although different, these children can adapt (Warren 1984). However, their development *is* different if only because they are seen as different by family and society. They also differ in experiencing through sound and touch which makes their development slower than sighted children who can exercise visual perception. Some blind children develop characteristic mannerisms known as 'blindisms' which depend on the lesion suffered, e.g. children with bilateral optic nerve defects never press their eyes (see below) whilst those with retinal disorders tend to press vigorously (Jan et al 1983). Outcome, in the absence of mental retardation, is good as eye pressing tends to fade (Freeman et al 1989).

Photophobia

Photophobia is seen in children with serious eye disease. Congenital glaucoma may cause photosensitivity due to abnormal corneal cells which are oedematous. Photophobia occurs in Leber's amaurosis and, if seen in the neonatal period, should be noted as this may be the only sign of this condition at this age.

Eye rubbing and pressing

Blind children are often seen eye-rubbing (Fig. 12.14). This is a distressing habit which, in older children who persistently eye press or poke (Fig.

manipulative tasks which require pre-timing (Henderson & Morris 1981).

- They experience difficulties in adapting their grip (Cole et al 1988).
- There are deficits in developing and utilizing pre-progammed motor sequences (Seyfort & Spreen 1979).
- The developmental sequence of postural reactions differs from non-handicapped babies (Haley 1987).

Malformations and other disabilities

Atlanto-axial instability occurs in 10–20% of children and there may be associated occipito-atlantal instability (Hungerford et al 1981), hypoplasia and other abnormalities in the craniocervical area. A rare hemiplegia due to atlanto-cervical dislocation has been recorded (Coria et al 1983). These malformations are due to congenital laxity of ligaments and Down syndrome children have difficulty in adjusting their heads in space (Rast & Harrias 1985). Other common disabilities are poor muscle tone, hearing loss, speech problems, strabismus and heart lesions.

Temperament

The original description by Down described the children as 'amiable and happy' and this stereotype has tended to remain but latterly this view has been questioned. They have temperaments which are 'easy', 'difficult' or 'slow-to-warm-up' i.e. similar to normal children (Huntington & Simeonsson 1987, Gunn et al 1981).

Institutions

Down syndrome children living in institutions do less well than those who live at home (Carr 1970, 1988).

Health problems

Poor health is a prominent feature of Down syndrome children. For example, in a study (Turner et al 1990) of 6–14-year-old children:

— 44% had a current *heart problem*, 7% of which were rated by their mothers as severe
— 70% had *visual defects* requiring treatment or follow-up
— 26% had a *continual hearing loss*
— 37% had a *variable hearing loss*
— 4% had *skin disorders*
— 68% had *respiratory problems* such as bronchitis, pneumonia, repeated

URTIs and asthma. Many children had three or more episodes of at least two different illnesses

— 24% had had three or more *throat infections* during the past year (compared with 13% of 7-year-olds in the NCDS)
— 88% had been *hospitalized* at some time during their life (45% for the 11-year-olds in the NCDS). Tonsillectomy, grommet insertion and squint correction were the most common operations.

These episodes of illnesses were associated with loss of school time, behavioural problems and maternal stress.

Follow-up

The implications are a continued need to follow these children and provide counselling service for their parents. The need for continued hearing tests is mentioned in Chapter 9.

Mortality

Mortality from leukaemia, other haemopoietic malignancies, congenital heart and other defects and chest infections are all higher than the whole population (Scholl et al 1982). Early signs of brain ageing similar to Alzheimer's disease have been described (Malamud 1972, Crapper et al 1975).

Intervention programmes

Whether highly structured (Barna et al 1980), unstructured (Cunningham et al 1977) or home-based (Woods et al 1984), early intervention programmes improve developmental quotients and minimize the progressive slowing of intellectual development. Parents' response to early intervention programmes has been little studied but Sloper et al (1983) noted that parents were, in general, positive about the programmes, finding the information supportive but the recording charts time-consuming.

CEREBRAL PALSY

Prevalence

In the South East Thames Regional Health Authority the prevalence of cerebral palsy, between 1970 and 1979, was 2.2 per 1000, 7.4% the result of multiple births. 58% were male. 35% weighed >2500 g and 8.5% were due to postnatal causes (Evans et al 1985). In Southampton, an incidence of 1.2 per 1000 births was recorded (Jones & Radford 1981). In Australia, the prevalence at age 6 was 3.6% for babies weighing less than 1500 g at birth and 4.3% for those weighing 1500–1999 g (Stanley & English 1986). Kiely et al (1981) concluded that there is no evidence for lowered or raised rates of cerebral palsy among surviving low-birthweight infants in recent years.

Types of cerebral palsy

Tables 13.9 and 13.10 show the distribution of types of cerebral palsy. Table 13.11 shows their impairments. It is thought that plasticity of the infant brain allows intact areas to take over the functions of damaged parts. Whilst this is to some extent true, early unilateral brain lesions can sometimes depress general cognition (James-Roberts 1981) and deficits suffered by unilateral brain lesions are more like those of adults than previously supposed. Hemiplegic cerebral palsied children, if examined

Table 13.9   Distribution of types of cerebral palsy (From Evans P, Elliott M, Alberman E, Evans S 1985 Prevalence and disability in 4–8 year olds with cerebral palsy. Archives of Disease in Childhood 60: 940–945, courtesy of the British Medical Association)

Diagnosis	Number	% of total number	% of those of known type
Dyskinetic	52	9.8	12.5
Spastic	270	51.2	64.7
Ataxic	39	7.4	9.4
Dyskinetic spastic	40	7.6	9.6
Dyskinetic ataxic	3	0.5	0.7
Ataxic spastic	13	2.5	3.1
Other types and type not known*	110	21.0	
Total	527	100	100

* The dyskinetic group includes choreoathetosis and dystonia; six cases were described only as 'hypotonic', but these are included under 'other types' as it was not clear how many had true hypotonic cerebral palsy.

Table 13.10   Distribution of subgroups described as spastic (From Evans P, Elliott M, Alberman, Evans S 1985 Prevalence and disability in 4–8 year olds with cerebral palsy. Archives of Disease in Childhood 60: 940–945, courtesy of the British Medical Association)

	Number	%
Hemiplegia	97	36
Diplegia	74	28
Quadriplegia	71	26
Monoplegia	6	2
Paraplegia	5	2
Other	17	6
Total	270	100

Table 13.11 Impairments by clinical type of cerebral palsy (From Evans P, Elliott M, Alberman E, Evans S 1985 Prevalence and disability in 4–8 year olds with cerebral palsy. Archives of Disease in Childhood 60: 940–945, courtesy of the British Medical Association)

	Ataxic		Spastic		Dyskinetic		Dyskinetic spastic		*All cases in study	
	Clinical form	(All cases)	Clinical form	(All cases)	Clinical form	(All cases)	Clinical form	(All cases)	Clinical form	(All cases)
Number of cases	32	(39)	191	(270)	34	(52)	28	(40)	332	(527)
Hearing(%)										
Severe defect	0	(0)	2	(2)	6	(4)	4	(2)	3	(2)
Moderate defect	3	(3)	6	(4)	6	(4)	4	(3)	6	(4)
Defect of unknown severity	0	(3)	4	(3)	0	(1)	0	(0)	1	(3)
No defect	97	(82)	88	(64)	82	(58)	92	(65)	87	(57)
Missing data	0	(12)	3	(27)	6	(33)	0	(30)	3	(34)
Vision(%)										
Severe defect	3	(3)	9	(8)	9	(6)	4	(2)	7	(6)
Moderate defect	6	(5)	17	(13)	15	(10)	18	(13)	16	(10)
Squint	19	(15)	17	(16)	17	(15)	32	(27)	19	(16)
Other defect, e.g. nystagmus	22	(21)	2	(3)	0	(0)	4	(3)	4	(4)
No defect	50	(46)	51	(36)	56	(38)	43	(30)	51	(33)
Missing data	0	(10)	4	(24)	3	(31)	0	(25)	3	(31)
Orthopaedic(%)										
Right hip defect	0	(0)	0	(0)	3	(4)	4	(2)	1	(1)
Left hip defect	0	(0)	2	(2)	6	(4)	4	(2)	2	(1)
Both hips	0	(0)	7	(5)	0	(2)	11	(8)	5	(3)
Other defect(s)	16	(13)	40	(32)	32	(23)	46	(33)	36	(26)
Hip(s) and 'other' defects	0	(0)	4	(3)	3	(2)	7	(5)	4	(3)
Defect(s) of unknown type	3	(5)	2	(4)	0	(2)	0	(10)	0	(4)
No defect	72	(59)	38	(27)	50	(34)	25	(18)	44	(28)
Missing data	9	(23)	7	(27)	6	(29)	3	(22)	6	(34)

* Includes cases for whom diagnostic type is not known, as well as cases in smaller diagnostic groups.

condition is the high incidence of mental retardation in siblings (Robinson 1986).

Prader–Willi syndrome

Approximately 50% of a wide sample of patients suffering from Prader–Willi syndrome have a chromosomal abnormality. The condition is thought to be genetically heterogeneous (Zellweger 1981). Children may present in babyhood with feeding difficulties but developmental delay is the more usual presentation to the DP. Obesity, which characterizes older children, is due to insatiable appetite, or rather not knowing when they are satiated. Behaviour problems are common (Greenswag 1987). Most die young of cor pulmonale (Laurance et al 1981).

Klinefelter's syndrome (47 XXY)

This syndrome is usually diagnosed late, possibly in adolescence. Ratcliffe et al (1982) found reduced testicular volume, gynaecomastia, decreased head circumferences and longer leg length compared with matched controls and affected boys had lower verbal scores on the WISC.

HYDROCEPHALUS AND SPINA BIFIDA

Neural tube defects are on the decline in the US and UK, a decline paralleled by an increase in antenatal screening. However, whilst antenatal screening is responsible for the decline in anencephaly it is yet not proven whether it accounts for the fall in prevalence of spina bifida (Stone 1987).

Physical handicaps

Two-thirds have severe physical handicaps and 18% require walking aids, 49% will be wheelchair-bound (Richards & McIntosh 1973).

Intelligence

61% of 100 children with spina bifida had IQs within the normal range (80–137) and 39% were below this range (Hunt 1981).

Behavioural problems

44% of children with operatively treated hydrocephalus had behavioural problems, irrespective of intelligence. The disturbances were a mixture of neurotic and antisocial disturbances and more common in boys (Connell & McConnel 1981). The school adjustment of spina bifida children, compared with non-disabled controls, was not noticeably different but they had significantly more emotional problems (Tew et al 1985).

Maternal age and previous fetal death

There is an increased risk of anencephaly and spina bifida with advanced maternal age and a previous fetal death (Strassburg et al 1983).

Siblings

Siblings of affected children are at greater risk of social problems (Nevin et al 1981) associated with socio-economic status. This was not confirmed by Strassburg et al (1983).

Limb malfunction

Children with myelomeningocele and hydrocephalus not only have lower limb malfunction but some problems in the upper limbs. Hand function, for example, was only 59% of normal in all the cases examined (Turner 1986). Cerebellar ataxia was the most common problem. Mobility is associated with upper limb abnormality, i.e. the more marked the neurological abnormality in the upper limb the less mobile the child (Wallace 1973).

School problems

Many start school late, attend part-time and an increasing number are in special schools as they grow older (Hunt et al 1985). Often school doctors do not have enough experience to counsel and advise the teachers.

Other problems

Spina bifida children have a variety of problems and handicaps and, for older children, incontinence may well be one of the worst. 64% of Hunt's 100 children had visual defects, 27% had epilepsy, 87% had suffered from accidents such as scalds, burns, fractures or pressure sores.

MENINGITIS

The sequelae or absence thereof appear to depend upon the age of onset, the causal agent and treatment (e.g. Swartz 1984, Feldman & Michaels 1988). Although the great majority of survivors are leading normal lives, a residual lower adaptive performance is the most commonly reported sequel (Sproles et al 1969, Sell et al 1972, Alon 1979). Infections in the neonatal period and first year of life, especially if accompanied by fits, carry the highest risk of ensuing damage. Small head circumferences,

Greenswag L R 1987 Adults with Prader-Willi syndrome: a survey of 232 cases. Developmental Medicine and Child Neurology 29: 145–152

Gunn G, Berry P, Andrews R J 1981 The temperament of Down's syndrome infants: a research note. Journal of Child Psychology and Psychiatry and Allied Disciplines 22: 189–194

Hagberg B, Edebol-Tysk K, Edstrom B 1988 The basic care needs of profoundly mentally retarded children with multiple handicaps. Developmental Medicine and Child Neurology 30: 287–293

Haley S M 1987 Sequence of development of postural reactions by infants with Down syndrome. Developmental Medicine and Child Neurology 29: 674–679

Harris M M, Dignam P F 1980 A non-surgical method of reducing drooling in cerebral-palsied children. Developmental Medicine and Child Neurology 22: 293–299

Hart R P, Henry G K, Kwentus J A, Leshner R T 1986 Information processing speed of children with Friedreich's ataxia. Developmental Medicine and Child Neurology 28: 310–313

Henderson S E, Morris J 1981 The motor deficit in Down's syndrome children: a problem of timing? Journal of Child Psychology and Psychiatry and Allied Disciplines 22:233–245

Herbert G W, Wilson H 1977 Socially handicapped children. Child: Care Health and Development 3: 13–21

Hersh J H, Bloom A S, Zimmerman A W et al 1981 Behavioral correlates in the Happy Puppet Syndrome: a characteristic profile? Developmental Medicine and Child Neurology 23: 792–800

Hertz R 1979 Retarded parents in neglect proceedings: the erroneous assumption of parental inadequacy. Stanford Law Review 31: 785–805

Hewson S, McConkey R, Jeffree D 1980 The relationship between structured and free play in the development of a mentally handicapped child: a case study. Child: Care, Health and Development 6: 73–82

Hinde R A 1980 Family influences. In: Rutter M (ed) Scientific foundations of developmental psychiatry. Heinemann, London

Hirst M 1984 After 16: the education of young people with special needs — a public campaign. The College Hill Press, Worthing

Hirst M 1985 Dependency and family care of young adults with disabilities. Child: Care, Health and Development 11: 241–257

Hirst M A 1983 Young people with disabilities: what happens after 16? Child: Care, Health and Development 9: 273–284

Ho H, Glahn T J, Ho J 1988 The fragile X syndrome. Developmental Medicine and Child Neurology 30: 252–265

Hoare P 1984a Psychiatric disturbance in the families of epileptic children. Developmental Medicine and Child Neurology 26: 14–19

Hoare P 1984b Does illness foster dependency? A study of epileptic and diabetic children. Developmental Medicine and Child Neurology 26: 20–24

Holt K 1958 The home care of severely retarded children. Pediatrics 22: 744–755

Holt K S 1975 The handicapped child. Child: Care Health and Development 1: 185–189

Howlin P 1988 Living with impairment: the effects on children of having an autistic sibling. Child: Care, Health and Development 14: 395–408

Hungerford G D, Akkaraju V, Rawe S E, Young G F 1981 Atlanto-occipital and atlanto-axial dislocations with spinal cord compression in Down's syndrome: a case report and review of the literature. British Journal of Radiology 54: 758–761

Hunt G M 1981 Spina bifida: implications for 100 children at school. Developmental Medicine and Child Neurology 23: 160–172

Huntington G S, Simeonsson R J 1987 Down's syndrome and toddler temperament. Child: Care, Health and Development 13: 1–11

James-Roberts L St 1981 A reinterpretation of hemispherectomy data without functional plasticity of the brain. Brain and Language 13: 531–532

Jeffery H, Scott J, Chandler D, Dugdale A E 1977 Deafness after bacterial meningitis. Archives of Disease in Childhood 52: 555–559

Jeffree D M, Cheseldine S E 1982 A new leisure class: the effect of training in leisure-time occupations on ESN(S) school leavers. Child: Care, Health and Development 8: 283–294

Jones C E M, Radford M 1981 Origin of handicap in young children. Archives of Disease in Childhood 56: 535–537

Jones M L 1985 Home care for the chronically ill or disabled child: a manual and sourcebook for parents and professionals. Harper & Row, London

Kahkonen M, Leisti J, Thoden C J, Autio S 1986 Frequency of rare fragile sites among mentally subnormal school children. Clinical Genetics 30: 234–238

Kayayama M, Tamas L B 1987 Saccadic eye-movements of children with cerebral palsy. Developmental Medicine and Child Neurology 29: 36–39

Kiely J L, Paneth N, Stein Z, Susser M 1981 Cerebral palsy and newborn care. II. Mortality and neurological impairment in low-birthweight infants. Developmental Medicine and Child Neurology 23: 650–659

Kiernan C 1977 Toward a curriculum for the profoundly retarded, multiply handicapped child. Child: Care, Health and Development 3: 229–239

King S M, Rosenbaum P, Armstrong R W, Milner R 1989 An epidemiological study of children's attitudes toward disability. Developmental Medicine and Child Neurology 31: 237–245

Ladda R L, Maisels M J, Dossett J H, Dobelle Y 1977 Chromosomal mosaicism in Down's syndrome: a diagnostic challenge. Developmental Medicine and Child Neurology 19: 668–672

Lademann A 1978 Postneonatally acquired cerebral palsy: a study of the aetiology, clinical findings and prognosis in 170 cases. Acta Neurologica Scandinavica 57: suppl 65

Lansdown R, Goldman A 1988 The psychological care of children with malignant disease. Journal of Child Psychology and Psychiatry and Allied Disciplines 29.5: 555–567

Laurance B M, Brito A, Wilkinson J 1981 Prader–Willi syndrome after age 15 years. Archives of Disease in Childhood 56: 181–186

Leibowitz D, Dubowitz V 1981 Intellect and behaviour in Duchenne muscular dystrophy. Developmental Medicine and Child Neurology 23: 577–590

Lejeune J, Gautheier M, Turpin R 1959 Les chromosomes humains en culture de tissus. Comptes Rendus de l'Academie des Sciences 248: 602–603

Lindsay J, Ounsted C, Richards P 1984 Long term outcome in children with temporal lobe seizures.V. Indications and contra-indications for neurosurgery. Developmental Medicine and Child Neurology 26: 25–32

Long C G, Moore J R 1979 Parental expectations for their epileptic children. Journal of Child Psychology and Psychiatry and Allied Disciplines 20: 299–312

Lonsdale G 1978 Family life with a handicapped child: the parents speak. Child: Care, Health and Development 4: 99–120

MacFaul R 1986 Medical care in severe mental handicap. Archives of Disease in Childhood 61: 533–535

MacKeith R C, Joseph M 1966 A New Look at Child Health. Pitman Medical, London

Malamud N 1972 Neuropathology of organic brain syndromes associated with aging. In: Gaitz C M (ed) Aging and the brain. Plenum Press, New York

Markova I, Forbes C 1979 Haemophilia: a study into social and psychological problems. Health Bulletin 37: 24–29

Markova I, MacDonald K, Forbes C 1980 Integration of haemophilic boys into normal schools. Child: Care, Health and Development 6: 101–109

Matthiessen C 1977 The development of equipment by the RCA. Child: Care, Health and Development 3: 43–48

McAndrew I 1976 Children with a handicap and their families. Child: Care, Health and Development 2: 213–237

McMichael J K 1971 Handicap: a study of physically handicapped children and their families. Staples Press, London

McQueen P C, Spence M W, Winsor E J T, Garner J B, Periera L H 1986 Causal origins of major mental handicaps in the Canadian maritime provinces. Developmental Medicine and Child Neurology 28: 697–707

Mearig J 1985 Facial surgery and an active modification approach for children with Down's syndrome: some psychological and ethical issues. Rehabilitation Literature 46: 72–77

Morss J R 1983 Cognitive development in the Down's syndrome infant: slow or different? British Journal of Educational Psychology 53: 40–47

Morss J R 1984 Enhancement of object-permanence performance in the Down's syndrome infant. Child: Care, Health and Development 10: 39–47

Moss P D 1982 Outcome of meningococcal group B. Meningitis 57: 616–621

Moyes C D 1980 Epidemiology of serious head injuries in childhood. Child: Care, Health and Development 6: 1–9

Newsom J, Newsom E 1979 Toys and playthings in development and remediation. Allen & Unwin, London

Placing developmental paediatrics within clinical medicine finds its most compelling justification because a wide range of developmental levels, abnormality and deviancy is recognized. The medical model allows interpretation of 'tests' in both application and performance. The psychometric view, by comparison, is of normal child development and the range of normality with retardation and superiority at the extreme points. (Psychometric 'tests', however, have the advantage of being standardized both in material and administration so are objective and have a baseline against which future measures can be matched.) The developmental view of diagnosis receives support from Piagetian theory. For example, in the psychometric view, a child with the *mental* age of 3 is the same whether his *chronological* age is 3 or 6 years. But in a developmental paediatric view a mentally retarded child aged 6, with a mental age of 3, will be 'locked' in the (Piagetian) sensorimotor stage whilst a normal 3-year-old will have moved to the pre-operational stage. The two children are developmentally different. The case for retaining of a medical model is also helped by the stability of cognition in abnormality. Whilst the influence of environment *can* alter performance, the change is insufficient to alter the prognosis. Cognitive achievements of a normally intelligent and Down syndrome child can be altered by living in an exceptionally deprived or highly stimulating environment, but the depression of functioning which severe deprivation produces in a normal child will not reach the level of severe mental retardation, whilst a highly stimulated Down syndrome child will never equal normality.

There are difficulties with a purely medical model. Personalsocial development, an extremely important parameter of human development which is less separate and discrete, is not included in these three subdivisions. Yet it, too, is subject to abnormalities, often affecting the other subdivisions especially A and C. Brain-damaged and mentally retarded children are more likely than normal children to have immature social development and suffer behavioural problems and all types of language problems have a strong association with psychiatric and social disturbance (Gualtieri et al 1983, Caulfield et al 1989). The reasons are both inherent and environmental. Personalsocial development is influenced by temperament type. Of the three temperament types described by Thomas & Chess (1977), the *difficult child* is more common in brain-damaged and mentally retarded children. The difficult type child is less amenable to environmental influences, being more distractible but rigid in thought process, and is likely to have an unsatisfactory mother/child relationship.

DEVELOPMENTAL DIFFERENTIAL DIAGNOSIS

The concept of differential developmental diagnosis has been described in Chapter 4. Levels in each developmental parameter, together with examination of hearing and vision, provide the basis upon which differential diagnosis is made. Development is normal, delayed or deviant in one or several parameters and deviancy can occur in all parameters. An example in motor development is a child with cerebral palsy who may roll from supine to prone before he has head control; an example in language development is the child who retains echolalia long after it normally disappears. Childhood psychoses are examples of deviant personalsocial development and specific learning difficulties of deviant learning. Table 14.1 shows a developmental differential diagnosis in some major developmental disabilities. It is assumed that the conditions are discrete, e.g. cerebral palsy or deafness are not accompanied by mental retardation, although, in practice, one handicap is often accompanied by another. It has to be decided which is the second handicap and how much it is affecting the developmental profile. Deafness is an example. It will not depress inherent cognition but affects achievement in different parameters to different degrees, nonverbal skills being less affected than linguistic ones: within the language parameter, if cognition is good, symbolic language is less affected than other subdivisions of language. Formal learning, depending upon intact verbal, nonverbal and perceptive skills, is affected but in different measures. Very high or low ability in any parameter is not necessarily reflected in other parameters. A child with an extremely high IQ does not usually have high personalsocial or motor development and may be a high myope or deaf.

McConachie et al (1989) outline some guidelines for the assessment of children with multiple handicaps and Illingworth (1987) describes 'pitfalls' in developmental diagnosis:

● Taking an inadequate history.
● Having a less than thorough knowlege of the average.
● Not taking ALL the factors which may affect developmental level into account.

Table 14.1   Differential diagnosis of major developmental disabilities

Developmental parameter	Language disorder	Mental retardation		Cerebral palsy	Deafness	Social deprivation
		Mild	Severe			
Motor						
Gross	N	N	V	D	N	N
Fine	N	MD	V	D	N	N
Adaptive	N	D	D	V	N	N or MD
Language						
Comprehension	D	D	D	N	D	N or MD
Expression	D	MD	D	D	D	MD
Symbolic	D	D	D	N	MD	N
Personal social	D	MD	D	V	N	MD

N = Normal; V = variable; D = delayed; MD = mildly delayed.

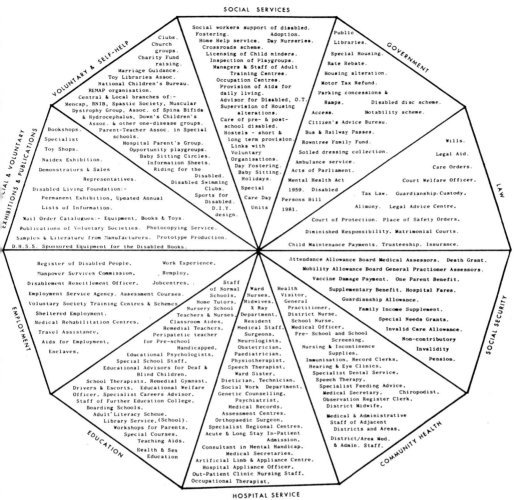

Fig. 14.1 Kaleidoscope showing the sources of answers to problems as guidance for handicapped children (From McGown MP 1982 Guidance for parent of a handicapped child. Child: Care, Health and Development 8:298. Prepared for the North East Thames Regional Paediatric Club Meeting, July 1981, by Dr M R McGown and Mr P Basham, courtesy of Blackwell Scientific Publications).

Doctors

Developmental paediatrician who retains infrequent but regular interviews with child and parents after diagnosis (see Ch. 13), often over years. Ballard (1978) has written how much this meant to him as a parent of a handicapped child but these interviews are useless unless the DP has a real relationship with parents and child. These interviews are more helpful if the home visitor accompanies mother and child to the appointment. The interview calls for a variety of skills from the DP, one of which is the ability to both understand and cope with aggression and negative reactions. MacKeith (1973) has written sensitively on the feelings and behaviour of parents of handicapped children. The inadequacy of many doctors (and others) in skills of communication has been noted (Wolraich & Reiter 1979). The interview includes examining physical, psychological and social aspects of the child and his family such as:

- physical and developmental reassessment of the child
- discussion with parents (and child) of the plan for continuing care and treatment
- the relationship of patient to his family and theirs towards him
- encouragement of parents and child in their coping skills
- sometimes nursery, school or residential placement.

Psychiatrist is skilled in behaviour problems which frequently accompany all types of disability. The diagnosis and treatment of autism is within his remit as is giving psychological support to other members of the Team and to special schools (Evered et al 1989).

Paediatric neurologist offers diagnosis, treatment and care to children suffering from damage to CNS, seizures in particular, and many motor problems.

Paediatric ophthamologist. The value of this doctor has been described in Chapter 12.

Orthopaedic surgeon diagnoses and treats many motor problems, advices on prostheses, aids etc.

Paediatric audiologist will diagnose and treat children with hearing problems and is responsible for hearing aids. He may visit deaf children in schools.

Community doctors have special skills in developmental paediatrics and are knowledgeable about and well-versed in using community social and educational resources. They visit schools, run the school medical service and often special clinics.

Psychologists may be clinical or educational.

Clinical psychologists have a degree in psychology and further training in clinical psychology. They are skilled in behavioural problems and disorders, behaviour modification, counselling and possibly psychotherapy. Their contribution in teaching behavioural therapy to other disciplines will be noted later.

Educational psychologists have often been teachers before taking a degree in educational psychology. Special education, school psychological problems and, sometimes, the assessment of learning difficulties is their expertise. They have personal knowledge of local schools and facilities and frequently liaise with and visit them.

The motor problem

The current motor problem depends on the age of the child. Retention of primitive reflexes and abnormal motor tone causes abnormal posture and the aim of physiotherapy is to reduce the latter. Tightness of the adductors may cause subluxation or dislocation of hip(s). Contractures and shortening of the tendo Achilles are a constant danger so sitting and standing in correct positions must be ensured. Chairs, splints, night orthoses, etc. may be required.

Deformities and contractures

An equinus deformity is the most common deformity and is treated with heel-cord lengthening, usually with good results. The varus deformity is more difficult to treat. Knee-flexion contractures are treated by passive stretching. Lengthening is by serial casting, splints or surgical treatment. Children with total body involvement, limited to lying in bed or sitting in a chair, develop secondary deformities such as scoliosis or hip dislocation which may be corrected by surgery and exercises (Bowen et al 1981). Katz et al (1988) suggested sitting rehabilitation by means of a seat insert should follow surgical correction. For treatment of scoliosis see later. Triple arthrodesis undertaken for hindfoot deformity and pain is best undertaken when the children are still walking (Ireland & Hoffer 1985). For optimistic views on treatment of cerebral palsy, Levitt's book on the subject is recommended (Levitt 1977). Motor developmental training; ways of helping the child in everyday functions; problems of deformity; equipment and therapeutic group work are all clearly described. Many less conventional types of treatment have been tried in this therapeutically frustrating condition. Some are more successful than others:

- one of the advantages of the Peto system (Cotton 1965) of conductive education is that therapist and teacher are the same person
- 'tone reducing' casts may be superior to standard casts in improving stride length (Hinderer et al 1988)
- music as a feedback mechanism to help head control (combined with a head position trainer) improved 3 of 5 severely mentally retarded cerebral palsied children
- rolfing technique involves pressure on areas where muscle tendons abnormally adhere to rather than slide over in the normal way and this has been used as a treatment in mildly impaired patients. The increased tightness of muscles outweighed any benefit gained in mobility (Perry et al 1981).

Second handicap

Approximately *one quarter* of children will have a hearing loss; *one in five* epilepsy and *half* mental retardation whilst visual and learning problems are extremely common. All require treatment and attention.

Everyday practical problems of handicapped children

Cerebral palsied children have frequent toileting and sleeping difficulties for which their parents need practical advice, e.g. information about local services such as a nappy service and how to apply for the attendance and mobility allowance.

Psychological and emotional problems

These are similar to those described earlier in this chapter. Cerebral palsy cannot be cured and parents tend 'to shop around'. Although understandable, the media sometimes does parents a disservice by making unreasonable claims of 'miracle' cures, e.g. the Delcato or the Peto system. The family doctor may be the best colleague whose help can be enlisted.

Cerebral palsy in adulthood

Apart from the normal needs of adults, Bleck (1984) has listed these as:
1. Equipment for efficiency and independence in daily life, e.g. computers, powered and other wheelchairs.
2. Surgery to relive pain and limit structural changes.
3. A programme of regular exercise.

How often are these objectives achieved?

Spina bifida

The management of children with spina bifida has gone through many changes in the past 30 years. An excellent summary of current therapy is available (McCarthy 1991).

Peritoneal catheter is a safer method of diverting CSF than the previously used atrial catheter; hydrocephalus is usually managed by ventriculoperitoneal shunt and neuropathic bladder by self-catherization. CAT scans can study shunt function. Paraplegics require devices to maintain ambulation. The treatment may be surgical and orthotic. Upper as well as lower limbs may have sensory deficits. Children with spina bifida require much medical input but not at the expense of normal stimulation so that emotional and cognitive growth does not become neglected. Assessment of spina bifida for educational placement calls for special insight and skills. The common association of visuospatial difficulties and 'cocktail party' language have been noted in other chapters.

25% have visual handicaps, usually strabismus. Babies selected for immediate surgery are likely to have a higher IQ than those in whom treatment is delayed (Tew et al 1985).

Duchenne muscular dystrophy

This condition is mentioned in preference to other motor disorders because of its fatal outcome which calls for different aspects of the care of patients and their families. Both have psychological needs which Taft (1973) defines as: making the diagnosis, offering genetic counselling and all the general aspects of long-term care. Expert psychiatric help is advisable early on especially if the affected child has seen another sibling affected. The children are likely to have repeated hospital admissions. Gait analysis is useful in measuring impairment and three gait patterns — early, transitional and late — have been described (Sutherland et al 1981). Quadriceps insuffiency is the key factor in gait deterioration and gait analysis will indicate when long-leg bracing is necessary to prolong ambulation. Ambulation has also been prolonged by lightweight knee-ankle-foot orthoses (Heckmatt et al 1985). Children should not become obese (Edwards et al 1984). Most are wheelchair-bound by 10 years.

Scoliosis

Scoliosis may occur in a number of neuromuscular diseases. Prevalence in cerebral palsy has been estimated at 15–38% (Bunnell & MacEwen 1977). It is a common and distressing feature of late Duchenne muscular dystrophy.

It may be treated by:

— seating system, e.g. the Toronto seat
— body braces when the curvature reaches 20°. There are different types and there is disagreement as to their efficacy. One type promotes a lordotic posture (Young et al 1984)
— plastic jackets (Bunnell & MacEwan 1977)
— surgical intervention stabilization can only be carried out if lung function is adequate and is recommended before the curve becomes 50° (Sussman 1985).

OTHER THERAPIES

Drugs

Epilepsy is the condition most often encountered in which drugs are commonly used and it is outside the scope of this book to describe these drugs in detail. For the DP it is important to establish (if possible) the exact diagnosis of the epilepsy because different drugs are more effective in different types of epilepsy. In general, the treatment of choice will be:

Grand mal epilepsy   – phenytoin
Focal epilepsy   – carbamezepine
Petit mal epilepsy   – ethosuximide
Temporal lobe epilepsy   – carbamezepine
Myoclonic epilepsy   – clonazepam
Infantile spasms   – ACTH or corticosteroids
Status epilepticus   – i.v. diazepam

There are alternatives for each type. All the drugs have side effects, drowsiness is the most common. Their relation to learning disabilities is discussed in Chapter 10. Even in the hands of experts, some fits prove intractable. The biggest debate is on the use of drugs in minimal cerebral dysfunction. This has been described in Chapter 6. Rarely, drugs are used in the control of obesity; a combination of diet and exercise intervention is more satisfactory. Weight loss is most satisfactory when attendance at an obesity clinic is accompanied by an exercise programme carried out at home (Hills & Parker 1988).

Diets

There is a limited place for the use of ketogenic diets in children with intractable seizures. Using medium-chain triclyceride diets, 81% of children with intractable seizures gained more than a 50% improvement in seizures (Swartz et al 1989). There was no evidence that artificial food colours were harmful when given to institutionalized children in a double-blind trial but neither was there improvement (Thorley 1984).

Mobility aids

The DP needs to know the underlying principles in the prescription of aids and appliances for handicapped children and three papers are compulsory reading: Blockey (1971), Barton et al (1980) and Holt (1991).

Motorized wheelchairs

Children with various disabilities were taught to use motorized wheelchairs. 50% improved in spatial exploration, interaction with objects and communication with caregiver, 33% improved in two spheres whilst the remainer only improved in spatial exploring (Butler 1986).

Hearing loss *see* Conductive hearing loss;
    Deafness; Sensorineural deafness
Hearing tests, 107, 131, 391–398
    1–5 years of age, 394–398
    and child's attention, 374
    for neonates, 392–394
    school children, 135
Heart disease, congenital, 350
Height, 22, 94, 95–97
    comparisons, 263
    weight ratio, malnutrition, 99, *fig. 4.6*
Hemiplegia
    draw-a-man test, 260, 261, *fig. 8.24*
    language development, 291
    locomotion milestone prediction,
        162–163, 169
    motor handicap, 171
    posture, 171, *fig. 6.18*
    spatial/verbal defects, 268
    strabismus association, 94, *fig. 4.2*
Hering theory, colour vision, 416
Heroard, 2
Hip, movements, 102–103
Hiskey-Nebraska scale of learning, 398
Historical aspects, 1–9
History-taking, 81–91, 117
    child, 82–89
    child/doctor relationship, 81, 82
    child/patient relationship, 81
    doctor/parent relationship, 81
    family life, 89–91
    parental memory, 81
    parents, 89–90
Holt, Kenneth, 5
Home and housing, 91
    and development, 58, 59, 61–62, 64
    high-rise flats, 61
Home visiting, and care, 531
    see also Health visitors
Homes, transitional, 537
Homocystinuria, 435
Hopping, 151
Hormone production, 24
Human figure, drawing 256–262,
    figs 8.18–8.25
    see also Draw-a-man test
Hunter syndrome, 93
Huntington's chorea, 509
Hurler syndrome, 93
Hydrocephalus, 88, 481–482
    language development, 291–292
    optic atrophy, 433
    see also Spina bifida
Hyperactivity, 178
    differences from clumsiness and mental
        retardation, 180–182
    management, 186–187
    presentation, 181
    prognosis, 183–184

Hypercalcaemia, idiopathic infantile, 93,
    269, 293
Hypermetropia, 40, 355
    IQ, 444
    neonatal, 414, 420, 423, 424, *fig. 12.7*
Hyperoxia, visual problems, 429, 432–433
Hypertonia, perinatal asphyxia, 49
Hypopituitarism, neonatal, 87
Hypothalamus, lesions, 24
Hypothyroidism, congenital, 69–70, 89, 96
    sensorineural deafness, 379
Hypotonia, 102
    blindness, 177
Hysteria, motor development effects,
    177–178

Illingworth, R. S., 5
Illinois Test of Psycholinguistic Abilities
    (ITPA), 267
Illness
    chronic, learning effects, 346
    and developmental stage, 42
    personal/social development, 214
Imitation, and learning, 326, 329, *fig. 10.4*
Immunological system, 24, 48
Impairment/disability/handicap, distinctions,
    506
Impulsiveness, adaptive development,
    264–265
Inattention, 340
    see also Attention
Infant motor screen, 167
Infantile spasms, 68, 86–87
Infection, resistance, 48
Ingestions/poisoning, and developmental
    stage, 41–42
Initial teaching alphabet (ITA), 360
Innumeracy, 352, 353, *fig. 10.15*
Insanity, and isolation, 195
Insecurity, 217
Instinctual (energy) drives (Freud), 12
Institutional upbringing, language
    development effects, 279, 290
Institutions, 536–537
Intelligence
    genetic/environmental factors, 66
    and learning, 343–344
    and socio-economic class, 64
    see also IQ
Intensive care units (ICUs), neonatal, 50, 52
Intention tremor, 101
Interim Hayes Binet test (IHB), 443
Interpretation, 30–33, *figs 2.5, 2.7*
Intrauterine maldevelopment, short stature,
    95
Invalid Children's Aid Association, 495
Investigations, 104–107
IQ
    and adaptive development tests, 242

IQ (*Cont'd*)
  epilepsy, 479
  mild/severe mental retardation, 522–523
  and play, 336
  spina bifida, 481
  visual defects, 444
IQ tests, 4, 38, 104–105
  low birthweight follow-up, 52
Iron deficiency anaemia, 69
Irradiation, and neoplasms, 68
Isle-of-Wight tests, 166
Isolation, and insanity, 195
Isotope brain scanning, 106

Jealousy, 205–206, 211–212, *fig. 7.10*
Jehuda ben Bezalee, 2
Jervell-Lange-Nielsen syndrome, 381
Joint sense, motor development, 164
Jumping, 150–151

Kemplex Tweeters, neonatal hearing test, 393
Kanner autism, 289, 295
Kearn syndrome, 435
Kernicterus, 384
Kinaesthesia, 160, 161, *fig. 6.12*
Klinefelter syndrome, 89, 97, 292, 481
Klippel-Feil syndrome, 93, 380
Kohs Block Design test, 443
Krabbe's disease, infantile, 512

Labyrinthine sense, 164
Lacerations, and developmental stage, 42
Ladder copying, 255, *fig. 8.16*
Landau-Kleffner syndrome, 286–287
Language
  and blindness, 289–290
  deaf-blind children, 289–290
  and deafness, 288–289, 290
  delays/disorders, 84
    intervention programmes, 307
    intervention timing, 306
    outcome, 538
    prevalence, 280–282
    and reading, 352
    signs/symptoms, 284–286
    social attachments, 211
    tests, 297–302
    treatment, 306–312
    types, 282–287
  see also Comprehension of language;
      Expressive language; Speech;
      Symbolic (inner) language
Language development, 33–37, 130–131, 276–322
  affecting factors, 278–280
  age sequences, 276–278
  cerebral palsy, 290–191
  child's sex, 278
  Chomsky, 275

chromosomal abnormalities, 292
comprehension delays/disorders, 282, 283–284
environment and demography, 279–280
environmental deprivation effects, 34, 36–37
expression delays/disorders, 282, 283
hemiplegia, 291
hydrocephalus, 291–292
and learning, 343, 353, 355
left hemisphere, 291
medical and developmental factors, 280
mental retardation, 290, 291
mixed delays/disorders, 282
nature/nurture aspects, 34, 36–37
parental role, 276, 278
and play, 335
and position in family, 278
psychological/psychiatric disorders, 294–296
school children, 134–135
and socio-economic class, 64, 279
spina bifida, 291–292
twins, 278
and visual defects, 447
Laterality, and learning, 343
Laughing, 203–204
Laurence-Moon-Biedl syndrome, 93, 96, 435
Lead poisoning, 70, 88–89
  visuospatial problems, 269
Learning, 37–38
  adaptive development, 242
  affecting factors, 337–350
  basic principles, 323
  drug therapy effects, 347–348
  environmental factors, 345–345
  medical factors, 345–350
  methods, 325–327
  Piagetian theory, 323–325
  school children, 135–136
  stages of reaction, 323–325
  and stimulation, early, 53–54
  theory, 12–13
Learning problems, 84, 347
  attention and concentration span, 356
  child profile, 356–357
  diagnosis, 357–359
  epilepsy, 479
  hearing testing, 355
  incidence, 350–351
  inheritability, 344
  investigations, 353–357, *fig. 10.16*
  language development test, 353, 355
  motor incoordination, 355–356
  nonverbal skills testing, 355
  testing, 351–357
  vision testing, 355
  visual/auditory perception, 355